NEPHROLOGY RESEARCH AND CLINICAL DEVELOPMENTS

KIDNEY TRANSPLANTATION

EFFICACY, SAFETY AND OUTCOMES

NEPHROLOGY RESEARCH AND CLINICAL DEVELOPMENTS

Additional books and e-books in this series can be found on Nova's website under the Series tab.

NEPHROLOGY RESEARCH AND CLINICAL DEVELOPMENTS

KIDNEY TRANSPLANTATION

EFFICACY, SAFETY AND OUTCOMES

ROBERT C. MORGAN
EDITOR

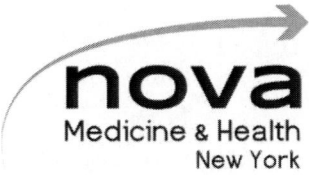

Copyright © 2021 by Nova Science Publishers, Inc.

All rights reserved. No part of this book may be reproduced, stored in a retrieval system or transmitted in any form or by any means: electronic, electrostatic, magnetic, tape, mechanical photocopying, recording or otherwise without the written permission of the Publisher.

We have partnered with Copyright Clearance Center to make it easy for you to obtain permissions to reuse content from this publication. Simply navigate to this **publication's** page on Nova's website and locate the "Get Permission" button below the title description. This button is linked directly to the title's permission page on copyright.com. Alternatively, you can visit copyright.com and search by title, ISBN, or ISSN.

For further questions about using the service on copyright.com, please contact:
Copyright Clearance Center
Phone: +1-(978) 750-8400   Fax: +1-(978) 750-4470   E-mail: info@copyright.com.

NOTICE TO THE READER

The Publisher has taken reasonable care in the preparation of this book, but makes no expressed or implied warranty of any kind and assumes no responsibility for any errors or omissions. No liability is assumed for incidental or consequential damages in connection with or arising out of information contained in this book. The Publisher shall not be liable for any special, consequential, or exemplary damages resulting, in whole or in part, from the readers' use of, or reliance upon, this material. Any parts of this book based on government reports are so indicated and copyright is claimed for those parts to the extent applicable to compilations of such works.

Independent verification should be sought for any data, advice or recommendations contained in this book. In addition, no responsibility is assumed by the Publisher for any injury and/or damage to persons or property arising from any methods, products, instructions, ideas or otherwise contained in this publication.

This publication is designed to provide accurate and authoritative information with regard to the subject matter covered herein. It is sold with the clear understanding that the Publisher is not engaged in rendering legal or any other professional services. If legal or any other expert assistance is required, the services of a competent person should be sought. FROM A DECLARATION OF PARTICIPANTS JOINTLY ADOPTED BY A COMMITTEE OF THE AMERICAN BAR ASSOCIATION AND A COMMITTEE OF PUBLISHERS.

Additional color graphics may be available in the e-book version of this book.

Library of Congress Cataloging-in-Publication Data

ISBN: 978-1-53619-721-1

Published by Nova Science Publishers, Inc. † New York

CONTENTS

Preface		**vii**
Chapter 1	Calcium – Phosphorus Metabolism and Mineral – Bone Disease after Kidney Transplantation *Jean J. Filipov and Emil P. Dimtrov*	**1**
Chapter 2	Psychosocial Assessment of the Live Kidney Donor and Recipient *Yasemin Kocyigit, Sanem Cimen and Ayse Gokcen Gundogmus*	**33**
Chapter 3	Donor Nephrectomy Techniques *Ahmet Emin Dogan, Sanem Guler Cimen, Tarik Kucuk and Sertac Cimen*	**61**
Chapter 4	Nephrectomy Timing for Polycystic Kidneys in Autosomal Dominant Polycystic Kidney Disease Patients Listed for Transplantation *Görkem Özenç, Sanem Guler Cimen and Sertac Cimen*	**83**
Index		**99**

PREFACE

Kidney transplantation is a medical procedure performed on patients with end-stage kidney disease that can increase their life expectancy by several years. However, the procedure involves some risk and potential complications. Chapter One of this monograph summarizes the current strategy for diagnosis and treatment of chronic kidney disease-associated mineral bone disease (CKD-MBD) in kidney transplant recipients and aims to demonstrate the latest findings and therapeutic options in the field beyond recent published guidelines. Chapter Two describes the necessity of involving a psychiatrist in the transplant team to facilitate positive outcomes in kidney transplants, as psychological factors can contribute to treatment non-compliance and other issues. Chapter Three defines the surgical techniques used in living donor nephrectomy, discusses the use and reliability of these techniques in different patient groups, and examines the long-term follow-up results of donors and recipients. Lastly, Chapter Four discusses the variables involved in treating patients with autosomal dominant polycystic kidney disease (ADPCKD), whose enlarged and deformed kidneys can complicate kidney transplantation.

Chapter 1 - Chronic kidney disease – associated mineral bone disease (CKD-MBD) is an important factor for higher morbidity and mortality in renal patients, due to diverse pathological abnormalities that affect not only bone health but encompass also cardiovascular pathology and biochemical changes. After successful kidney transplantation (KT) a significant improvement in calcium-phosphorus metabolism occurs. However, moderate to advanced CKD persists in significant proportion of the kidney transplant recipients (KTRs). What is more, transplant-specific factors contribute to marked post-transplant CKD-MBD: immunosuppressive agents, sun avoidance, post-transplant diabetes mellitus, etc. Thus, different abnormalities in this cohort of patients can be detected, leading to poorer survival compared to the general population. The aim of the authors' study is to summarize the current strategy for diagnosis and treatment of CKD-MBD in KTRs and to demonstrate the latest findings and therapeutic options in the field beyond the recent published guidelines, in an attempt to offer solutions for improvement in post-transplant outcomes.

Chapter 2 - Chronic diseases provoke various psychological and behavioral problems and thus necessitate psychiatric evaluation. One of the most common chronic diseases worldwide is chronic kidney disease. The best treatment method for chronic kidney disease is a live donor kidney transplantation. However, it requires a healthy person, the donor, to undergo a surgical procedure for the sake of a loved one. Unfortunately, after the transplant procedure, poor outcomes related to non-compliance can be recorded in varying ratios. Treatment non-compliance may lead to chronic allograft rejection and loss of the donated kidney. In many cases, an in-depth psychological evaluation can predict adverse post-transplant events such as non-compliance and propose improvement strategies. Therefore, the inclusion of a psychiatrist in the transplant team helps to prevent these undesirable outcomes. When the recipient, living donor, along with their family decides to proceed with the transplant, it is a lifelong commitment. A favorable psychiatric evaluation for both the donor and recipient is a testimony of all participants` willingness and commitment to the best outcome. This review highlights common issues faced at different stages of this lengthy pathway.

Chapter 3 - Renal transplantation from a living donor has better results than cadaveric renal transplantation in terms of patient and graft survival rate, quality of life, and cost. Renal transplantation from living donors is performed safely with positive results due to insufficient cadaveric renal supply. The most classic and commonly used donor nephrectomy technique is the open technique performed with a flank lumbotomy incision. Today, this technique has been rapidly replaced by minimally invasive laparoscopic or robot-assisted donor nephrectomy techniques. This study aims to define the surgical techniques used in living donor nephrectomy, discuss the use and reliability of these techniques in different patient groups, and examine the long-term follow-up results of donors and recipients. There was no significant difference in complication rates, cost-effectiveness, and graft function in patients undergoing laparoscopic donor nephrectomy compared to open donor nephrectomy. On the other hand, renal transplantation centers should offer donors a few different techniques according to their needs and unique circumstances. Laparoscopic donor nephrectomy has become the gold standard technique for suitable living kidney donors in the last decade. However, it should be kept in mind that open, retroperitoneoscopic, robotic, and hand-assisted techniques can be safely applied for donor nephrectomy in the presence of donor-specific risk or limiting factors such as a history of previous abdominal surgery, multiple kidney arteries or veins, or obesity.

Chapter 4 - Autosomal dominant polycystic kidney disease (ADPCKD) is a common hereditary disorder causing end-stage renal disease in approximately 10% of the population worldwide. Its symptoms occur in the third and fourth decades of life, due to kidney enlargement and deformation, subsequently leading to renal failure. The definitive treatment of ADPCKD does not exist and current treatment regimens focus on managing the symptoms. For end-stage renal disease, the best treatment, providing a higher quality of life and overall survival is kidney transplantation. Kidney transplant outcomes are even better with live kidney donations. With live kidney donors, the timing of transplant can be planned and variables can be adjusted to achieve optimal conditions. One of these variables is caused by enlarged and deformed kidneys. These enlarged kidneys may trouble the transplant process by intra-cystic bleeding, infections, stone formations, and mechanical compression of other organs. Additionally, when enlarged below the iliac crest, these kidneys may occupy the space needed for the transplanted kidney. Thus, management of the polycystic kidneys at the pre-transplant period is curial. The decision to remove them, whether to remove single or both kidneys, and the timing of this surgery may affect the outcome of the kidney transplantation significantly.

In: Kidney Transplantation
Editor: Robert C. Morgan

ISBN: 978-1-53619-721-1
© 2021 Nova Science Publishers, Inc.

Chapter 1

CALCIUM – PHOSPHORUS METABOLISM AND MINERAL – BONE DISEASE AFTER KIDNEY TRANSPLANTATION

Jean J. Filipov[*]*, PhD and Emil P. Dimtrov*
*Department of Nephrology and Transplantology,
Hospital Lozenetz, Sofia, Bulgaria*

ABSTRACT

Chronic kidney disease – associated mineral bone disease (CKD-MBD) is an important factor for higher morbidity and mortality in renal patients, due to diverse pathological abnormalities that affect not only bone health but encompass also cardiovascular pathology and biochemical changes. After successful kidney transplantation (KT) a significant improvement in calcium-phosphorus metabolism occurs. However, moderate to advanced CKD persists in significant proportion of the kidney transplant recipients (KTRs). What is more, transplant-specific factors contribute to marked post-transplant CKD-MBD: immunosuppressive agents, sun avoidance, post-transplant diabetes mellitus, etc. Thus, different abnormalities in this cohort of patients can

---

[*] Corresponding Author's E-mail: jeanphillipov@yahoo.com.

be detected, leading to poorer survival compared to the general population. The aim of our study is to summarize the current strategy for diagnosis and treatment of CKD-MBD in KTRs and to demonstrate the latest findings and therapeutic options in the field beyond the recent published guidelines, in an attempt to offer solutions for improvement in post-transplant outcomes.

Keywords: chronic kidney disease, kidney transplantation, calcium-phosphorus metabolism, mineral bone disease

1. Introduction

Significant pathological changes occur in calcium-phosphorus (CaP) metabolism in patients with chronic kidney disease (CKD). These encompass not only biochemical abnormalities, but also bone health and vascular pathology, which significantly increase morbidity and mortality in renal patients. After successful kidney transplantation (KT) a rapid improvement in CaP metabolism takes place. However, the outcomes after KT are modified due to pre- and post-transplant factors. The aim of our chapter is to demonstrate the well-known post-transplant CaP changes and to evaluate the recent findings in mineral bone disease after KT.

2. Role of the Kidney in Calcium-Phosphorus Metabolism: Healthy Subjects

CaP homeostasis is regulated by bone, intestines and kidneys. Intestinal calcium and phosphorus absorption are enhanced by calcitriol and parathyroid hormone (PTH). Bones are the largest calcium deposit in human body. Elevated PTH and metabolic acidosis increase calcium bone resorption, whereas calcitonin reduces calcium levels by suppressing the osteoclasts [1]. Other hormonal factors (estrogens, androgens, etc) also play a significant role in regulating CaP metabolism.

The kidneys participate actively in CaP homeostasis via CaP filtration and tubular handling. Calcium filtration is enhanced in increased renal blood flow and glomerular filtration pressure. Calcium reabsorbtion in the renal tubules is stimulated by PTH, higher serum phosphate, metabolic/respiratory acidosis, calcitriol. It should be noted, that diuretics influence calcium renal excretion too. Loop diuretics and mannitol reduce calcium renal reabsorption, whereas thiasides and amiloride increase it [2]. Phosphate is reabsorbed in the proximal tubules. The resorption is promoted by calcitriol and is suppressed by PTH, increased extracellular volume. A key factor, enhancing phosphate excretion is fibroblast growth factor 23 (FGF-23). FGF-23 was detected as one of the most important phosphatonins in the body. Apart from phosphate homeostasis, this bone-derived hormone probably causes left vehtricular hypertrophy and is involved in vascular calcification in CKD patients. Other promoters of phosphate excretion are soluble α klotho and FGF-7 were also detected. The importance of phosphatonins in CKD, especially FGF-23 will be discussed later.

A key renal function is the synthesis of 1,25 – dihydroxyvitamin D (1,25VD or calcitriol) in the renal tubules. 1,25VD is the most active vitamin D metabolite, that influences CaP metabolism via the vitamin D receptor (VDR). In the kidneys the last hydroxylation of vitamin D occurs, transforming it into active molecule. As VDRs were detected in many organs, a mechanism of action of 1,25VD, spanning beyond CaP homeostasis (VD pleiotropy) was suggested.

3. Calcium-Phosphorus Metabolism in Chronic Kidney Disease (CKD). CKD-Related Mineral Bone Disease (MBD)

Chronic kidney disease (CKD) is defined as decreased estimated glomerular filtration rate (eGFR) below 60 ml/min/1,73m^2 or the presence of albuminuria, urine sediment abnormalities, electrolyte and other abnormalities due to tubular disorders, pathology detected by histology, disorders detected by imaging or history of kidney transplantation [3]. CKD affects CaP metabolism and causes significant deterioration of bone and cardiovascular health, leading to increased mortality and morbidity in CKD patients. CKD – associated CaP pathology combines laboratory findings, bone disorders and vascular pathology and is referred to CKD-associated mineral bone disease (CKD-MBD).

3.1. Pathophysiology

The loss of functioning nephrons causes reduction in phosphate excretion. The initial hyperphosphatemia is the primary step in CaP disorder in CKD. However, at the initial CKD stages phosphate levels are maintained within normal range until eGFR of approx. 35 ml/min/1,73m^2 is reached due to the activation of the phosphaturic hormones FGF-23 and PTH [2]. In addition to increased phosphaturia, FGF-23 suppresses the transformation of 25-hydroxyvitamin D to calcitriol. Apart from influencing CaP metabolism, FGF-23 causes left ventricular hypertrophy and transformation of smooth muscle cells within the vascular wall to osteoblasts, enhancing calcium deposits and vascular disease in CKD patients [4, 5]. Similar to phosphate, calcium levels are preserved within normal level until more advanced CKD stages are reached. Though total body calcium is reduced due to calcitriol synthesis suppression, normal calcium level is supported by elevated PTH and increased osteoclast activity. Vitamin D (VD) metabolism is severely affected too: not only calcitriol synthesis is suppressed, but also its precursors' formation is reduced (due to uremic skin, reduced sun exposure, protein dietary restrictions etc.), as well as downregulated VDR expression and dysfunction were also detected [6].

Parathyroid gland abnormalities play a pivotal role in CKD. Hypocalcemia and hyperphosphatemia directly stimulate PTH synthesis. However, lower VD levels and poorer VDR expression in the parathyroid tissue also contribute to additional stimulation of the gland. Reduced expression of calcium-sensing receptors and parathyroid gland hyperplasia further complicate CKD-related hyperparathyroidism, which is a main therapeutical target in renal disease. Finally, alkaline phosphatase (ALP), both total (tALP) and bone-specific (bALP), which is elevated in primary and secondary hyperparathyroidism, reflects higher bone turnover.

The pathophysiological changes described above lead to CKD-related mineral bone disease (CKD-MBD), which has 3 aspects: biochemical abnormalities, bone disease and vascular disorders.

3.2. CKD-MBD: Biochemical Abnormalities

The major laboratory indicators that are being evaluated in CKD-MBD are serum calcium, phosphate, PTH and ALP activity, and is recommended to start as soon as eGFR below 60 ml/min/1,73m^2 is detected. According to Kidney Disease Improving Global Outcomes (KDIGO) the frequency monitoring is suggested to be performed according to the CKD stage and the magnitude of abnormalities [7]. The following frequencies were suggested by KDIGO in the latest guidelines:

- eGFR 59 – 30 ml/min/1,73m^2: serum calcium and phosphate, every 6–12 months; and for PTH, based on baseline level and CKD progression.
- eGFR 29 – 15 ml/min/1,73m^2: serum calcium and phosphate, every 3–6 months; and for PTH, every 6–12 months.
- eGFR below 15 ml/min/1,73m^2: serum calcium and phosphate, every 1–3 months; and for PTH, every 3–6 months.
- In CKD stages 4 and 5, including patients on dialysis: for alkaline phosphatase activity, every 12 months, or more frequently in the presence of elevated PTH.

More frequent testing can be performed when therapy is being performed in order to evaluate the effect from therapy and avoid side effects [7]. KDIGO also recommends initial evaluation of VD status, once

CKD is diagnosed, by measuring serum 25-hydroxyvitamin D (25VD), rather than calcitriol levels. FGF-23 is not tested routinely due to the use of different testing methods and lacking standardization. In addition, lowering FGF-23 has not demonstrated improvement in outcomes in CKD patients, though higher levels were associated with poorer patient survival [8].

The major therapeutic goals are lowering of serum phosphate, normalization of calcium levels, (special attention is paid to avoiding hypercalcemia) and correction of PTH and correction of vitamin D deficiency [7]. Inadequate therapy of hyperparathyroidism and CaP abnormalities can cause serious complications (e.g., adynamic bone disease), that may influence post-transplant outcomes. Therefore, special attention should be paid to the correction of CKD-MBD biochemical parameters. The latest KDIGO guidelines suggest that KT should not be performed until secondary hyperparathyroidism is adequately corrected [9].

3.3. CKD-MBD: Bone Disease

Bone involvement in CKD-MBD is associated with higher prevalence of fractures and higher mortality in the adult CKD population. Factors, influencing fracture risk are age, gender (females), presence of diabetes, use of steroids and longer dialysis treatment. Bone health is evaluated by assessing PTH and bone ALP levels, as well as bone mineral density (BMD). In addition, KDIGO suggests bone biopsy in the evaluation of CKD- related bone disease, if the information obtained will have impact on treatment strategy [7].

There are 3 histological indicators that determine 5 types of bone disorder in CKD: bone turnover, mineralization and bone volume. Bone turnover (T) corresponds to bone formation rate. It can be abnormally low, normal, or very high and is best assessed via bone biopsy and tetracycline labelling. Mineralization (M) is measured by osteoid maturation time and mineralization lag time and is classified as normal and abnormal. Bone volume (V) demonstrates bone formation and resorption rates. It is defined as low, normal, and high. Thus, the TMV classification is formed, with the following 5 types of renal osteodystrophy defined [10]:

a) Adynamic bone disease (AD): low-turnover bone disease with normal mineralization. Volume can be low, but in some cases it can be normal. AD is often due to iatrogenic PTH oversuppression
b) Mild secondary hyperparathyroidism related bone disease (MHPTBD): medium to high bone turnover, any bone volume, normal mineralization
c) Osteitis fibrosa (OF): a more advanced form of high-turnover disease, compared to MHPT, any bone volume, normal mineralization
d) Osteomalacia (OM): low-turnover bone with abnormal mineralization. Bone volume may be low to medium, depending on the severity and duration of the process
e) Mixed uremic osteodystrophy (MUO): represents features of the above-mentioned variants; for example, a combination of high-turnover, normal bone volume, with abnormal mineralization.

In addition, bone pathology due to osteoporosis (age-related/postmenopausal) can be detected. Finally, normal histology may also be established; its prevalence is higher in CKD patients not on dialysis (approx. 16%), whereas on hemodialysis or peritoneal dialysis its prevalence drops to 2% [11]. Histological findings are influenced by different factors: malnutrition, inadequate CKD-MBD treatment, presence of diabetes, age. Type of dialysis treatment is also of great importance, as the prevalent bone disorder in patients on peritoneal dialysis is AD [11]. Dialysis duration is an independent factor increasing fracture risk [12]. Therefore, timely KT would be the best option in CKD patients requiring renal replacement therapy, as it would reduce the risk for CKD-MBD complications.

Bone biopsies are the golden standard for histological evaluation. However, they are not performed routinely, as they are painful, laborious, time-consuming, and expensive. Indications for the procedure are bone fractures, bone pain, unexplained hypercalcemia/hypophosphatemia, evaluation of the type of bone turnover (which may lead to treatment correction), and suspected aluminum toxicity [7, 13]. According to the 2017 KDIGO guidelines bone biopsy is not indicated prior anti-resorptive therapy in CKD, as this treatment causes significant reduction of fracture incidence in CKD patients, without evidence for AD induction. Nevertheless, bisphosphonates should be used with caution in CKD and CKD-MBD should be addressed first [7]. Generally, excessively elevated PTH and bone-specific ALP can be used in clinical practice to predict bone turnover in CKD-MBD. Two types of CKD-MBD have been defined: high turnover mineral bone disease (HTMBD) and low turnover mineral bone disease (LTMBD). In most cases the two entities cannot be differentiated clinically from each other, laboratory findings play a key role in the differential diagnosis (Table 1). In cases, in which clinical and laboratory data are inconclusive of the type of bone turnover, bone biopsy should be considered [7].

Table 1. High turnover MBD vs low turnover MBD – laboratory and histological differentiation

Indicator	HTMBD	LTMBD
Serum calcium	N in early stages ↓/N/↑ (advanced)	early stages N/↑ advanced stages - ↑↑
Serum phosphate	N in early stages N to very high (advanced)	early stages N/↓ advanced stages - ↓/↑
BAP	N in early stages ↑ in advanced HTMBD	early stages N/↓ advanced - ↓
PTH	N/↑ in early stages ↑↑↑ (advanced)	early stages N/↓ advanced stages ↓
Histology	OF, MHPTBD	AD, OM

HTMBD – high turnover mineral bone disease, LTMBD – low turnover mineral bone disease, PTH – parathyroid hormone, BAP – bone specific alkaline phosphatase, N – normal, ↓ - decreased, ↑ - increased values, OF – osteitis fibrosa, MHPTBD - mild secondary hyperparathyroidism related bone disease, AD – adynamic bone disease, OM – osteomalacia.

The association between the type of renal osteodystrophy (ROD) and fracture risk is uncertain, as some studies demonstrate increased fracture risk in certain types (especially AD), whereas others do not support this association [7, 14]. In addition, AD linked to higher rate of vascular calcification; CKD patients with LTMBD were also found to have higher risk for coronary artery calcifications [15, 16]. Furthermore, the shift from HTMBD to LTMBD after parathyroidectomy contributed to progression to vascular calcification [17]. After successful KT a rapid decrease in bone mineral density occurs, increasing additionally the fracture risk [18]. Therefore, adequate treatment of pre-transplant CKD-MBD is mandatory in order to improve posttransplant outcomes.

3.4. CKD-MBD: Vascular Involvement

Vascular calcification (VC) can be detected in up to 93% and valvular calcification is found in 20 – 47% of the dialysis patients [19, 20]. CKD-MBD associated vascular involvement affects typically the muscular layer of medium or large arteries and can be diagnosed by using CT scan, but lateral abdominal radiograph and echocardiogram can be used as alternative diagnostic tools; different scoring methods, such as computer tomography coronary artery calcification score and Kauppila scoring have been suggested to quantify VC in renal disease [21]. CKD patients with vascular pathology are considered to be at highest risk for cardiovascular events [7]. Treatment of vascular/valvular calcification has two aspects: treatment of CKD-MBD and atherosclerosis.

3.4.1. CKD-MBD

Correction of hyperphosphatemia proved to be important factor for VC progression. Most of the studies demonstrate faster VC progression when calcium binders are used, compared to sevelamer treatment [22, 23]. The effect from cholecalciferol/calcitriol supplementation on VC is not fully elucidated. Generally, lower 25VD and 1,25VD are associated with VC progression. However, higher doses of cholecalciferol/calcitriol can worsen VC [24, 25]. The role of vitamin D analogues (VDA) in VC progression also remains unclear. Though initially VDAs were detected to cause milder VC, compared to calcitriol treatment, a recent study failed to establish any benefit from paricalcitol in VC progression compared to calcitriol [26, 27]. Finally, the current body of evidence demonstrates a possible beneficial effect on VC from calcimimetics in animal models; however, the results have not been fully confirmed in humans, therefore the current guidelines do not support calcimimetics' use for improving patient survival and improving cardiovascular outcomes only [28].

3.4.2. Atherosclerosis

Pharmacological treatment of atherosclerosis in CKD has demonstrated unclear benefit. The current KDIGO guideline recommends statin /statin+ezetimibe treatment in patients with CKD not on dialysis. In dialysis dependent patients however the benefits from initiating antilipid treatment are insignificant, therefore it should not be initiated. In contrast to the dialysis cohort, in kidney transplant recipients antilipid treatment can be initiated, as it significantly improves cardiovascular outcomes after KT [29].

4. POST-TRANSPLANT CALCIUM-PHOSPHORUS METABOLISM AND MBD

4.1. Post-Transplant Calcium – Phosphorus Metabolism: Pathophysiology and Biochemical Abnormalities

After successful KT, due to the presence of functioning nephrons and elevated FGF-23, a rapid increase of phosphaturia follows. This results in a rapid decrease in phosphate serum levels, which in turn leads to rapid decrease of FGF-23 after KT [30]. Furthermore, the presence of active nephrons improves VD metabolism as the new functioning tubules enhance the synthesis of the active VD metabolite 1,25-dihydroxyvitamin

D. However, negative post-transplant trends in CaP metabolism are also present, mainly due to persistent poorer graft function and secondary hyperparathyroidism. Up to 70% of the KTRs were found to have eGFR lower than 60 ml/min/1,73m2, explaining the widely detected CKD-related abnormalities, whereas secondary hyperparathyroidism was detected in 39% of the post-transplant cases 4 years after KT [31, 32].

4.1.1. Vitamin D

VD metabolism is impaired due to persistent CKD after KT, as well as transplant-specific factors: sun avoidance, the prevalence of post-transplant diabetes, higher obesity rates, and use of immunosuppressive agents. For instance, steroids enhance VD catabolism, whereas calcineurin inhibitors are associated with VD deficiency, as they interfere with 25VD liver synthesis [33]. Our results clearly demonstrate high prevalence of VD insufficiency, especially in the autumn – winter fall.

VD's influence on mineral-bone metabolism has been extensively evaluated. Current findings demonstrate, that cholecalciferol supplementation effectively lowers PTH levels, without significant prevention of bone loss [34]. However, a large study has demonstrated that cholecalciferol supplementation reduces fracture risk; yet, more studies are needed to evaluate the influence of VD on post-transplant fracture incidence [35]. In addition, its pleiotropic (extraskeletal) effects are currently a hot topic in transplantology. The concept of VD pleiotropy is based on the widely detected VDR and the presence of nonrenal 1-α hydroxylase. Several extraskeletal properties were reported: renin – angiotensin - aldosterone system suppression, renal protection, antiproteinuric effects, immunomodulatory properties, improved diabetes control, reduced cancer and infection risk in *in vitro* models, animal studies, in the general population and CKD patients. It could be speculated, that VD status optimization can reduce rejection incidence, infection and neoplastic risk, and improve cardiovascular health, thus improving post-transplant graft and patient survival. In our transplant center we have established higher proteinuria and higher risk for cancer in poorer VD status in KTRs [36, 37]. Observational studies have demonstrated, that poorer VD status was linked to higher post-transplant mortality and faster GFR decline; beneficial effect from VD analogues treatment on proteinuria was also detected [38, 39]. Unfortunately, VD pleiotropy after KT is still under debate due to the small, single – center trials, reporting controversial results.

4.1.2. Calcium, Phosphate, PTH

Steroids suppress intestinal calcium reabsorption and cause steroid-induced ostheoporosis. In addition, PTH levels remain elevated after kidney transplantation due to persistent parathyroid hyperplasia, that may cause hypercalcaemia [32]. After successful KT, hypophosphatemia can be detected in up to 86% of the KTRs, with its peak detected 16.5 days post-transplant, with rapid improvement in phosphate levels afterwards [40]. In this study several risk factors for hypophosphatemia [females, younger recipient and donor age, lower body mass index (BMI), higher post-transplant eGFR, lower panel reactive antibody (PRA) result] and for hypercalcemia (males, younger KTRs, higher BMI, higher graft eGFR, longer duration of dialysis) were detected. However, calcium and phosphate levels were poor predictors of graft survival and mortality.

It should be noted, that biochemical abnormalities can be influenced by the presence of CKD stage 3 or higher. Thus, a complex laboratory post-transplant constellation is present, requiring individualized approach in every patient.

4.1.3. Monitoring and Treatment of CaP Abnormalities

Immediately after KT calcium and phosphate levels are being tested at least once weekly, until stable levels are achieved. After stabilization the frequency of monitoring is based on the magnitude of the abnormalities, the rate of CKD progression. Generally, KDIGO suggests similar to native CKD post-transplant monitoring and correction of CaP abnormalities. Cinacalcet can be used for the treatment of post-transplant hypercalcemia and persistent secondary hyperparathyroidism. However, this treatment has no effect on post-transplant BMD [41]. Oral phosphate supplementation should be used in severe hypophosphatemia (phosphorus < 0.64 mmol/L) [18].

Testing for 25VD should be performed after KT and further testing should be based on baseline values and treatment. Vitamin D supplementation should follow the strategies designed for the general population [7].

4.2. Post-Transplant Calcium – Phosphorus Metabolism: Bone Disease

Post-transplant bone disease (PTBD) is associated with abnormal bone density and quality, which coupled with abnormal post-transplant mineral metabolism leads to higher fracture risk and higher mortality after KT. Generally, BMD declines in the early post-transpant period. Its decline slows down afterwards; however, it remains lower than the general population. These changes lead to higher fracture risk than the general population even 10 years after successful KT. The most common sites for fracture are the hip and ankle/foot [42].

Table 2. Risk factors for post-transplant bone disease (PTBD)

Pre-transplant	Post-transplant
Females	Cumulative steroid dose
Older age	Vitamin D insufficiency
Malnutrition	Persistent hyperparathyroidism
BMI < 23	
Smoking, alcohol	
Poor physical activity	
Diabetes mellitus	
CKD-MBD	
Duration of dialysis	
Hypogonadism	

BMI – body mass index, CKD-MBD – chronic kidney disease – associated mineral bone disease.

Compared to dialysis patients, the risk is higher during the first 3 years after KT and lower thereafter [43]. Since 2010 a trend for lower fracture incidence is present, probably due to lower cumulative steroid dose and better treatment of pre-transplant CKD-MBD [42]. Several risk factors for PTBD have been identified, classified as pre-transplant and post-transplant ones (Table 2) [44].

4.2.1. Diagnosis and Fracture Risk Evaluation

4.2.1.1. Bone Mineral Density (BMD)

The use of dual energy X-ray absorptiometry (DXA) is limited due to its inability to differentiate trabecular from cortical bone (differently affected in CKD-MBD) and the fact that steroid - induced fractures are detected at higher BMD than in non-steroid induced ones [18]. Yet, several studies have demonstrated DXA to be reliable tool in fracture risk evaluation, especially BMD testing of the hip across all stages of CKD, including KTRs [45–47]. Therefore, the current KDIGO guidelines recommend the use of BMT testing in all post-transplant CKD categories, in KTRs with risk factors for osteoporosis, if this will alter therapy [7]. A typical frequency of DXA monitoring is immediately after KT and every 2 years thereafter, though other intervals are also possible [46].

4.2.1.2. FRAX Score

The FRAX score is a tool, evaluating the 10 – year risk for major fracture in the general population. Factors such as age, gender, BMI, family history of fracture, alcohol use, smoking, steroid treatment, history of rheumatoid arthritis, data for secondary osteoporosis (due to diabetes mellitus, liver disease, hypogonadism, hyperparathyroidism, premature menopause, chronic malnutrition/malabsorption) and BMD are incorporated in the risk-evaluation calculator. However, the tool has some disadvantages, most important of which is the missing CKD as parameter in the calculation. Recent studies have demonstrated, that FRAX score can be effective predictor for fracture risk both in native CKD and after KT

[18, 48]. Larger clinical trials are needed to evaluate the predictive value of the tool after kidney transplantation.

4.2.1.3. Bone Biopsy

Despite the directly obtained information for bone health by bone biopsy, the procedure is rarely performed in KTRs as well as in native CKD due to the limited centers that can evaluate the specimen, the discomfort during the procedure and the difference in the findings in different regions of the body [18]. Post-transplant bone biopsy studies so far have established a poor association between bone turnover markers and bone histology, as well as increasing incidence of low turnover bone disease [13]. The 2017 KDIGO guidelines suggest bone biopsy if it will influence therapy, referring to the more liberal approach in native CKD and the relatively safe profile of antiresorptive agents in CKD[7].

4.2.1.4. Bone Turnover Markers (BTMs)

Different turnover markers have been tested in the general population and CKD as predictors of fracture and their association with BMD. The most commonly evaluated ones are bALP, tALP, PTH, procollagen type I N propeptide (P1NP), C-terminal cross-linking telopeptide of type I collagen (CTX), tartrate-resistant acid phosphatase-5b (TRAP-5b) and urine deoxypyridinoline (uDPD). Most of these have limited importance in CKD due to thei renal excretion. There is a limited number of studies evaluating the predictive value of BTMs after KT. PTH, bALP, P1NP and TRAP5b failed to predict post-transplant fracture incidence, though inverse correlation between BTMs and BMD was detected [47]. A recent study also discovered similar correlation between P1NP, bALP and post-transplant BMD; however, fracture risk was not evaluated [49]. Due to the controversial results BTMs are not widely used as fracture predictors in KTRs.

4.2.1.5. Other Tools

High-resolution peripheral quantitative computed tomography (HRpQCT) is a relatively new technique, assessing bone microstructure and bone density of trabecular/cortical bone. HRpQCT effectively detected post-transplant BMD loss [42, 50]; however, studies evaluating its predictive role for fracture risk and comparison to DXA after KT are lacking, thus limiting its use in practice.

4.2.2. Treatment of Post-Transplant Bone Disease

4.2.2.1. Calcium, Phosphate, Vitamin D Supplementation/Calcitriol/Vitamin D Analogues

Post-transplant calcium levels are corrected as in native CKD. As already mentioned, hypophosphatemia is corrected at levels lower that 0.64 mmol/L. However, too aggressive phosphate supplementation may worsen secondary hyperparathyroidism and cause nephrocalcinosis, therefore normalization of phosphate levels should be avoided.

VD insufficiency is widely reported in KTRs. The current guidelines suggest that VD insufficiency is corrected as in the general population. Courbebaisse et al. demonstrated, that high doses vs low doses of cholecalciferol demonstrate significant reduction in fracture incidence without causing hypercalcemia, hyperphosphatemia or vascular calcification [35]. It should be noted that in this trial the high doses arm received 100000 IU cholecalciferol, whereas the low dose arm – 12000IU, both arms at the following intervals: every two weeks for two months, then monthly for the next 22 months. The low dose arm practically received a maintenance dose of 400 IU/daily, corresponding to the lower threshold for VD supplementation in the general population [51]. Therefore, despite the current guidelines, we can expect that higher doses of cholecalciferol than generally suggested may be needed after KT.

Treatment with calcitriol or VDA has also demonstrated improvement in BMD, PTH and bone turnover markers [39]. However, the use of these preparations bears the risk for hypercalcemia and hyperphosphatemia, especially taking the presence of pre-transplant CKD-MBD into consideration [18]. Thus, the abnormal levels of PTH, calcium, phosphate, ALP and 25VD should influence the treatment strategy in KTRs [7].

4.2.2.2. Calcimimetics

Cinacalcet is a drug that activates the calcium-sensing receptor in parathyroid cells, thus inhibiting PTH secretion and lowers serum calcium due to suppression of PTH-dependent calcium release from bone and increase of calcium renal loss. Though its use is not approved for the treatment of CKD-MBD after KT, the drug was successfully used to control secondary hyperparathyroidism and correct hypercalcemia and hypophosphatemia in KTRs [52]. Unfortunately, after stopping treatment PTH, calcium and phosphate levels quickly return to pre-treatment levels. In addition, no improvement in BMD after post-transplant cinacalcet treatment was established [53]. Thus, calcimimetics' use is limited in renal transplantation.

4.2.2.3. Antiresorptive Therapy: Bisphosphonates

Bisphosphonates inhibit osteoclastic bone resorption. Their use in native CKD is increasing due to the better understanding of their benefit: risk ratio. After successful KT, bisphosphonates prevented or improved low BMD in KTRs, without causing allograft dysfunction. The data for fracture risk reduction are limited: only one review demonstrated mild decrease in the fracture incidence in post-transplant bisphosphonate use [54, 55]. In addition, treatment with pamidronate was associated with increased risk for adynamic bone disease [56]. Thus, bisphosphonate treatment in CKD stages 1T – 3T (eGFR $\geq$ 30 ml/min/1,73m^2) should take into consideration the CKD-MBD biochemical abnormalities and bone histology if needed. The experience with bisphosphonates in CKD stages 4T – 5T and after the first year post-transplant is limited [7].

4.2.2.4. Antiresorptive Therapy: Denosumab

Denosumab is a human monoclonal antibody, binding with hig specificity to the receptor activator of nuclear factor κB ligand (RANkB-L), thus blocking RANkB – dependent osteoclast formation and activation, which in turn leads to reduction in bone resorption and improvement in BMD. Denosumab has demonstrated beneficial effect on BMD in KTRs [50]. In addition, it proved to be superior to bisphosphonates after KT, with slightly elevated risk for hypocalcemia [57]. Other side effects detected was increase urinary tract infections' rate [7]. Finally, Denosumab treatment discontinuation was associated with worsening of BMD in KTRs, similarly to pre-transplant CKD [58].

4.2.2.5. PTH Analogues

Teriparatide is a PTH analogue, which effectively improves BMD in steroid-dependent osteoporosis by stimulating bone formation. In KTRs however, it failed to demonstrate significant benefit on BMD loss, which coupled with its high cost limit significantly its use after KT [59].

4.2.2.6. Parathyroidectomy

Parathyroidectomy (PTX) is invasive procedure, preserved for the cases of persistent hyperparathyroidism and hypercalcemia, which are not medically controlled, as well as in complications from hypercalcemia, such as renal stone disease and nephrocalcinosis. It is generally performed at least 12 months after KT, as within this period post-transplant PTH level reduction is expected. Compared to cinacalcet, PTX effectively decreased calcium and PTH levels in KTRs, with improvement in femoral BMD, without significant changes in allograft GFR the two arms [60, 61]. The possible complications are hypocalcemia, failure to achieve adequate PTH control, recurrent laryngeal nerve injury.

4.2.2.7. Other Therapeutic Options

Steroid minimization or withdrawal caused improvement in BMD and fracture risk, without significantly increasing the risk for rejection. However, steroid discontinuation should be considered in KTRs with low immunological risk.

Other treatment options suggested in the general population and possibly effective in CKD are cessation of smoking, alcohol intake reduction, treatment of malnutrition, regular physical activity (reducing fall incidence), and vitamin K supplementation [62, 63]. Finally, in KTRs with all stages of post-transplant CKD and low BMD, treatment of CKD-MBD should follow the guidelines suggested for CKD patients not on dialysis [7].

4.3. Post-Transplant Calcium – Phosphorus Metabolism: Vascular Calcification

4.3.1. Diagnosis and Clinical Importance of Post-Transplant VC

Cardiovascular disease (CVD) is a leading cause of death post-transplant, with estimated prevalence up to 55% of all cases of death with functioning graft [64]. The presence of VC is directly linked to CVD after KT. VC, evaluated by coronary artery calcification (CAC) or aortic calcification (AoC) was detected in 60 to 75% KTRs [65]. Basically, the same diagnostic methods for detection and evaluation of post-transplant VC are being used, as in pre-transplant CKD. Several risk factors for post-transplant VC progression have been identified: age of the recipient, time on dialysis, magnitude of calcification/CKD-MBD, presence of diabetes, vitamin D status, immunosuppressive agents (steroids, calcineurin inhibitors), graft function, blood pressure [65]. A recent study identified age of recipient, calcification score at baseline, higher systolic blood pressure and use of Tacrolimus as additional risk factors for VC progression [66]. A possible explanation for the negative impact of immunosuppressive agents (steroids and calcineurin inhibitors) on vascular health is their effect on bone health and biochemical paramethers.

4.3.2. Treatment of Post-Transplant VC

As already mentioned, a significant improvement in renal function and biochemical paramethers after successful KT occurs, which are key factors for VC in CKD. However, recent findings demonstrate, that AoC and CAC progression can slow down, but VC does not regress in the post-transplant period, which can explain the higher mortality and CVD incidence in KTRs compared to the general population [67]. Thus, adequate treatment of pre-transplant CKD-MBD has a pivotal role in vascular health after renal transplantation.

4.3.2.1. Immunosuppression

Steroids and calcineurin inhibitors can worsen vascular health by suppressing the production of nitrogen oxide. Mycophenolate moefetyl and rapamycin inhibited smooth muscle cell proliferation, whereas everolimus impaired the antithrombotic function of endothelial cells [65]. Therefore, we can expect, that by carefully managing immunosuppresive regimen we can at least partially influence the progression of vascular pathology.

4.3.2.2. Vitamin D Supplementation

Observational studies have established association between lower 25VD and VC. Interventional studies however do not demonstrate improvement in CVD outcomes after high doses VD were applied in KTRs [35]. Thus, the effectiveness of VD supplementation in post-transplant VC progression remains unclear.

4.3.2.3. Other Therapeutic Options

Okamoto et al. demonstrated, that alendronate treatment halted the progression of AoC in KTRs. Unfortunately, the study encompassed a small number of patients (n = 12) [68].

Recently, the role of vitamin K in bone and vascular health has been demonstrated. Vitamin K is involved in the carboxylation of vascular Matrix Gla Protein, thus inhibiting arterial calcification. A recent prospective trial established lower incidence of coronary heart disease in Vitamin K2 supplemented patients [69]. Unfortunately, though observational studies have detected vitamin K deficiency in renal disease, interventional trials targeting CKD patients are lacking [70].

Raggi et al. showed that treatment with intravenous myo-inositol hexaphosphate (SNF472) effectively attenuated CAC and aortic valce calcification in hemodialysis patients [71]. It can be speculated, that similar effect can be detected in other CKD cohorts, including KTRs.

Finally, it should be noted, that VC may not be the adequate therapeutic target, as it constitutes disease marker and prognostic factor, rather than a cause for CVD. Therefore, trials evaluating different interventions and their effect on clinical outcomes may be more relevant for clinical practice [72].

CONCLUSION

Post-transplant calcium-phosphorus metabolism and mineral bone disease have significant impact on patient survival after renal transplantation. Randomized trials, evaluating the correct end-points and new therapies are needed. However, as current post-transplant interventions have controversial results, adequate pre-transplant treatment of CKD-MBD plays a pivotal role. In addition, shorter time on dialysis could provide healthier vascular and bone background after KT.

REFERENCES

[1] Guyton, A.; Hall, J., ed. 2000. Parathyroid Hormone, Calcitonin, Calcium and Phosphate metabolism, Vitamin D, Bone and Teeth. In: *Textbook of Medical Physiology*, 10 th. 899 – 914. W. B. Saunders.

[2] Kestenbaum, B., Drüeke, T. B. 2010. Disorders of Calcium, Phosphate, and Magnesium Metabolism In: *Comprehensive Clinical Nephrology*. Edited by Richard J. Johnson, Jürgen Floege and John Feehally. Fourth edi. 123 – 141. Saunders Elsevier.

[3] KDIGO. 2013. "Official Journal of the International Supplements Society of Nephrology KDIGO 2012 Clinical Practice Guideline for the Evaluation and Management of Chronic Kidney Disease." *Kidney International Supplements* 3, no. 1: 136–50.

[4] Stöhr, R., Schuh, A., Heine, G. H., and Brandenburg, V. 2018. "FGF23 in Cardiovascular Disease: Innocent Bystander or Active Mediator?" *Frontiers in Endocrinology*. doi:10.3389/fendo.2018. 00351.

[5] Jimbo, R., Kawakami-Mori, F., Mu, S., Hirohama, D., Majtan, B., Shimizu, Y., Yatomi, Y., Fukumoto, S., Fujita, T. and Shimosawa, T. 2014. "Fibroblast Growth Factor 23 Accelerates Phosphate-Induced Vascular Calcification in the Absence of Klotho Deficiency." *Kidney International* 85 (5): 1103–11. doi:10.1038/ki.2013.332.

[6] Filipov, J. J., and Dimitrov, E. P. 2017. "Vitamin D after Kidney Transplantation: Metabolism and Clinical Importance." *EMJ Nephrol.* 5 (1): 75–82.

[7] KDIGO. 2017. "Clinical Practice Guideline for the Diagnosis, Evaluation, Prevention and Treatment of Chronic Kidney Disease Mineral and Bone Disorder (CKD-MBD)." *Kidney International Supplements* 76 (Suppl 113): S1–128. doi:10.1038/ki.2009.188.

[8] Bouma-de Krijger, A., and Vervloet, M. G. 2020. "Fibroblast Growth Factor 23: Are We Ready to Use It in Clinical Practice?" *Journal of Nephrology.* 33(1): 509 - 527 doi:10.1007/s40620-020-00715-2.

[9] Chadban, S. J., Ahn, C., Axelrod, D. A., Foster, B. J., Kasiske, B. L., Kher, V., Kumar, D., et al. 2020. "KDIGO Clinical Practice Guideline on the Evaluation and Management of Candidates for Kidney Transplantation." *Transplantation* 104 (4S1 Suppl 1): S11–103. doi:10.1097/TP.0000000000003136.

[10] Moe, S., Drüeke, T., Cunningham, J., Goodman, W., Martin, K., Olgaard, K., Ott, S., Sprague, S., Lameire, N., and Eknoyan, G. 2006. "Definition, Evaluation, and Classification of Renal Osteodystrophy: A Position Statement from Kidney Disease: Improving Global Outcomes (KDIGO)." *Kidney International.* doi:10.1038/sj.ki. 5000414.

[11] Parfitt, A. M. 2003. "Renal Bone Disease: A New Conceptual Framework for the Interpretation of Bone Histomorphometry." *Current Opinion in Nephrology and Hypertension.* doi:10.1097/ 00041552-200307000-00007.

[12] Wetmore, J. B., Liu, J., Wirtz, H. S., Gilbertson, D. T., Cooper, K., Nieman, K. M., Collins, A. J., and Bradbury, B. D. 2016. "Geovariation in Fracture Risk among Patients Receiving

Hemodialysis." *Clinical Journal of the American Society of Nephrology* 11(8): 1413–21. doi:10.2215/CJN.11651115.

[13] Evenepoel, P., D'Haese, P., Bacchetta, J., Cannata-Andia, J., Ferreira, A., Haarhaus, M., Mazzaferro, S., Proust, Marie-Helene Lafage, Salam, S., Spasovski, G. and Cozzolino, M. 2017. "Bone Biopsy Practice Patterns across Europe: The European Renal Osteodystrophy Initiative - A Position Paper." *Nephrology Dialysis Transplantation.* doi:10.1093/ndt/gfw468.

[14] Carbonara, C. L. M., Quadros, K. R., Roza, N. A., Sano, R., Carvalho, A. B., Jorgetti, V., and de Oliveira, R. B. 2020. "Renal Osteodystrophy and Clinical Outcomes: Data from the Brazilian Registry of Bone Biopsies - REBRABO." *Jornal Brasileiro de Nefrologia: 'Orgao Oficial de Sociedades Brasileira E Latino-Americana de Nefrologia* 42 (2): 138–46. doi:10.1590/2175-8239-JBN-2019-0045. [*Brazilian Journal of Nephrology: Official Body of Brazilian and Latin American Nephrology Societies*]

[15] Barreto, D. V., Barreto F. C., de Carvalho A. B., Cuppari L., Draibe S. A., Dalboni M. A., Moyses R. M., Neves, K. R., Jorgetti, V., Miname, M., Santos, R. D. and Canziani, Maria Eugênia F. 2008. "Association of Changes in Bone Remodeling and Coronary Calcification in Hemodialysis Patients: A Prospective Study." *American Journal of Kidney Diseases* 52 (6): 1139–50. doi:10.1053/j.ajkd.2008.06.024.

[16] London, G. M., Marty C., Marchais S. J., Guerin A. P., Metivier F., and De Vernejoul M. C. 2004. "Arterial Calcifications and Bone Histomorphometry in End-Stage Renal Disease." *Journal of the American Society of Nephrology* 15 (7): 1943–51. doi:10.1097/01.ASN.0000129337.50739.48.

[17] Hernandes, F. R., Canziani, M. E., Barreto, F. C., Santos, R. O., De Melo, M. V., Rochitte, C. E., and Carvalho, A. B. 2017. "The Shift from High to Low Turnover Bone Disease after Parathyroidectomy Is Associated with the Progression of Vascular Calcification in Hemodialysis Patients: A 12-Month Followup Study." *PLoS ONE* 12 (4). doi: 10.1371/journal.pone.0174811.

[18] Vangala, C., Pan, J., Cotton, R. T., and Ramanathan, V. 2018. "Mineral and Bone Disorders after Kidney Transplantation." *Frontiers in Medicine.* 5: 1-16. doi:10.3389/fmed.2018.00211.

[19] Oh, K. W., Nam, C. M., Jee, S. H., Choe, K. O., and Suh, I. 2002. "Coronary Artery Calcification and Dietary Cholesterol Intake in Korean Men." *Acta Cardiologica* 57 (1): 5–11. doi:10.2143/AC.57.1.2005372.

[20] Ix, J. H., Shlipak, M. G., Katz, R., Budoff, M. J., Shavelle, D. M., Probstfield, J. L., Takasu, J., Detrano, R., and O'Brien, K. D. 2007. "Kidney Function and Aortic Valve and Mitral Annular Calcification in the Multi-Ethnic Study of Atherosclerosis (MESA)." *American Journal of Kidney Diseases* 50 (3): 412–20. doi:10.1053/j.ajkd.2007.05.020.

[21] Nelson, A. J., Raggi P., Wolf M., Gold A. M., Chertow G. M., and Roe M. T. 2020. "Targeting Vascular Calcification in Chronic Kidney Disease." *JACC: Basic to Translational Science.* doi:10.1016/j.jacbts.2020.02.002.

[22] Russo, Domenico, C. S., Miranda, I., Ruocco, C., Manzi, S., Elefante, R., Brancaccio, D., Cozzolino, M., Biondi, M. L., and Andreucci, V. E. 2007. "Progression of Coronary Artery Calcification in Predialysis Patients." *American Journal of Nephrology* 27 (2): 152–58. doi:10.1159/000100044.

[23] Barreto, Daniela V., Barreto, Fellype De Carvalho, De Carvalho, A. B., Cuppari, L., Draibe, S. A., Dalboni, M. A., Moyses, R. M. A., Neves, K. R., Jorgetti, V., Miname, M., Santos, R. D. and Canziani, Maria Eugênia F. 2008. "Phosphate Binder Impact on Bone Remodeling and Coronary Calcification - Results from the BRiC Study." *Nephron - Clinical Practice* 110 (4). doi:10.1159/ 000170783.

[24] Schlieper, Georg, Schurgers, L. Brandenburg, V., Reutelingsperger, C., and Floege, J. 2016. "Vascular Calcification in Chronic Kidney Disease: An Update." *Nephrology Dialysis Transplantation.* 31(1):31-39doi:10.1093/ndt/gfv111.

[25] Zhou, J. H., Wang, Y. M., Harris, D. C., Medbury, H., Williams, H., Durkan, A. M., Elder, G., et al. 2015. "High Dose Vitamin D-Induced Accelerated Vascular Calcification Is Associated with Arterial Macrophage Infiltration and Elevation of TLR4 Expression." *Nephrology* 20: 31.

[26] Zand, Ladan, and Kumar, R. 2017. "The Use of Vitamin D Metabolites and Analogues in the Treatment of Chronic Kidney Disease." *Endocrinology and Metabolism Clinics of North America*. 46(4): 983 – 1007. doi: 10.1016/j.ecl.2017.07.008.

[27] Anis, Karim H., Pober, D., and Rosas S. E. 2020. "Vitamin D Analogues and Coronary Calcification in CKD Stages 3 and 4: A Randomized Controlled Trial of Calcitriol versus Paricalcitol." *Kidney Medicine* 2 (4): 450–58. doi: 10.1016/j.xkme.2020.05.009.

[28] Lim, Kenneth, Hamano, T., and Thadhani, R. 2018. "Vitamin D and Calcimimetics in Cardiovascular Disease." *Seminars in Nephrology*. 38(3): 251–266. doi: 10.1016/j.semnephrol.2018.02.005.

[29] Kidney Disease Improving Global Outcomes (KDIGO) Lipid Work Group. 2013. "Clinical Practice Guideline for Lipid Management in Chronic Kidney Disease." *Kidney International* 3 (3): 259–305.

[30] Prasad, Narayan, Jaiswal, A., Agarwal, V., Kumar, S., Chaturvedi, S., Yadav, S., Gupta, A., Sharma, R. J., Bhadauria, D., and Kaul, A. 2016. "FGF23 Is Associated with Early Post-Transplant Hypophosphataemia and Normalizes Faster than iPTH in Living Donor Renal Transplant Recipients: A Longitudinal Follow-up Study." *Clinical Kidney Journal* 9 (5): 669–76. doi:10.1093/ckj/sfw065.

[31] Marcén, Roberto, Morales, J. M., Fernández-Rodriguez, A., Capdevila, L., Pallardó, L., Plaza, J. J., Cubero, J. J., Puig, J. M., Sanchez-Fructuoso, A., Arias, M., Alperovich, G., and Serón, D. 2010. "Long-Term Graft Function Changes in Kidney Transplant Recipients." *NDT Plus* 3 (SUPPLL. 2). doi:10.1093/ndtplus/sfq063.

[32] Filipov, J. J., Zlatkov, B. K., Dimitrov, E. P., and Svinarov, D. 2015. "Relationship between Vitamin D Status and Immunosuppressive Therapy in Kidney Transplant Recipients." *Biotechnology and*

Biotechnological Equipment 29 (2). doi:10.1080/13102818.2014.995 415.

[33] Filipov, J. J., Petrova, M., Metodieva, T., Dimitrov, E. P., and Svinarov, D. 2018. "Vitamin D Influences the Prevalence of Non-Cutaneous Carcinomas after Kidney Transplantation?" *Biotechnology & Biotechnological Equipment*, June, 1–5. doi:10.1080/13102818.2018.1482233.

[34] Messa, Piergiorgio, Regalia, A, and Alfieri, C. M. 2017. "Nutritional Vitamin D in Renal Transplant Patients: Speculations and Reality." *Nutrients*. doi:10.3390/nu9060550.

[35] Courbebaisse, Marie, Alberti, C., Colas, S., Prié, D., Souberbielle, J. C., Treluyer, J. M., and Thervet, E. 2014. "VITamin D Supplementation in renAL Transplant Recipients (VITALE): A Prospective, Multicentre, Double-Blind, Randomized Trial of Vitamin D Estimating the Benefit and Safety of Vitamin D3 Treatment at a Dose of 100,000 UI Compared with a Dose of 12,000 UI." *Trials* 15 (1): 430. doi:10.1186/1745-6215-15-430.

[36] Filipov, J. J, Zlatkov, B. K., Dimitrov, E. P. and Svinarov, D. 2016. "Higher 25-Hydroxyvitamin D Levels Are Associated With Lower Proteinuria in Kidney Transplant Recipients." *Experimental and Clinical Transplantation* 14 (6): 629–33. doi:10.6002/ect.2015.0344.

[37] Muirhead, N., Zaltman, J. S., Gill, J. S, Churchill, D. N., Poulin-Costello, M., Mann, V., and Cole, E. H. 2014. "Hypercalcemia in Renal Transplant Patients: Prevalence and Management in Canadian Transplant Practice." *Clinical Transplantation* 28 (2): 161–65. doi:10.1111/ctr.12291.

[38] Keyzer, Charlotte A., Riphagen, Ineke J., Joosten, M. M., Navis, G., Muller, Kobold A. C., Kema, Ido P., Bakker, Stephan J. L., and De Borst, Martin H. 2015. "Associations of 25(OH) and 1,25(OH)2 Vitamin D with Long Term Outcomes in Stable Renal Transplant Recipients." *Journal of Clinical Endocrinology and Metabolism* 100 (1): 81–89. doi:10.1210/jc.2014-3012.

[39] Trillini, Matias, Cortinovis, M., Ruggenenti, Piero, Loaeza, J. R., Courville, K., Ferrer-Siles, C., Prandini, S., Gaspari, F., Cannata, A.,

Villa, A., Perna, A., Gotti, E., Caruso, M. R., Martinetti, D., Remuzzi, G., and Perico, N. 2014. "Paricalcitol for Secondary Hyperparathyroidism in Renal Transplantation." *Journal of the American Society of Nephrology: JASN* 26: 1–10. doi:10.1681/ASN.2013111185.

[40] Chevarria, J., Sexton, D. J., Murray, S. L., Adeel, C. E., O'Kelly, P., Williams, Y. E., O'Seaghdha, C. M., Little, D. M., and Conlon, P. J. 2020. "Calcium and Phosphate Levels after Kidney Transplantation and Long-Term Patient and Allograft Survival." *Clinical Kidney Journal*. doi:10.1093/ckj/sfaa061.

[41] Delos, Santos R., Rossi, A., Coyne, D., and Maw, T. T. 2019. "Management of Post-Transplant Hyperparathyroidism and Bone Disease." *Drugs* 79 (5): 501–13. doi:10.1007/s40265-019-01074-4.

[42] Bouquegneau, Antoine, Salam, S.Delanaye, P., Eastell, R., and Khwaja, A. 2016. "Bone Disease after Kidney Transplantation." *Clinical Journal of the American Society of Nephrology*. doi:10.2215/CJN.11371015.

[43] Drüeke, Tilman B., and Evenepoel, P. 2019. "The Bone after Kidney Transplantation." *Clinical Journal of the American Society of Nephrology*. doi:10.2215/CJN.04940419.

[44] Kovvuru, K., Kanduri, S. R., Vaitla P, Marathi R, Gosi S, Garcia, Anton D. F., Cabeza Rivera, F., and Garla, V. 2020. "Risk Factors and Management of Osteoporosis Post-Transplant." *Medicina (Lithuania)*. doi:10.3390/medicina56060302.

[45] West, Sarah L., Lok, C. E., Langsetmo. L., Cheung, A. M., Szabo, E, Pearce, D., Fusaro, M., Wald, R., Weinstein, J., and Jamal, S. A. 2015. "Bone Mineral Density Predicts Fractures in Chronic Kidney Disease." *Journal of Bone and Mineral Research* 30 (5): 913–19. doi:10.1002/jbmr.2406.

[46] Akaberi, S., Simonsen, O., Lindergård, B., and Nyberg, G.. 2008. "Can DXA Predict Fractures in Renal Transplant Patients?" *American Journal of Transplantation* 8 (12): 2647–51. doi:10.1111/j.1600-6143.2008.02423.x.

[47] Evenepoel, P., Claes, K., Meijers, B., Laurent, M. R., Bammens, B., Naesens, M., Sprangers, B., Pottel, H., Cavalier, E., and Kuypers, D. 2019. "Bone Mineral Density, Bone Turnover Markers, and Incident Fractures in de Novo Kidney Transplant Recipients." *Kidney International* 95 (6): 1461–70. doi: 10.1016/j.kint.2018.12.024.

[48] Whitlock, Reid H., Leslie, W. D., Shaw, J., Rigatto, C., Thorlacius, L., Komenda, P., Collister, D., Kanis, J. A., and Tangri, N. 2019. "The Fracture Risk Assessment Tool (FRAX®) Predicts Fracture Risk in Patients with Chronic Kidney Disease." *Kidney International* 95 (2): 447–54. doi: 10.1016/j.kint.2018.09.022.

[49] Heimgartner, N., Graf, N., Fre,y D., Saleh, L., Wuthrich, R. P., and Bonani, M. 2020. "Predictive Power of Bone Turnover Biomarkers to Estimate Bone Mineral Density after Kidney Transplantation with or without Denosumab: A Post Hoc Analysis of the POSTOP Study." *Kidney and Blood Pressure Research* 45 (5): 758–67. doi:10.1159/000510565.

[50] Bonani, M, Frey, D., Graf, N., and Wüthrich, R. P. 2019. "Effect of Denosumab on Trabecular Bone Score in de Novo Kidney Transplant Recipients." *Nephrology Dialysis Transplantation* 34 (10): 1773–80. doi:10.1093/ndt/gfy411.

[51] Amrein, K, Scherkl, M., Hoffmann, M., Neuwersch-Sommeregger, S., Köstenberger, M., Berisha, A. T., Martucci, G., Pilz, S, and Malle, O. 2020. "Vitamin D Deficiency 2.0: An Update on the Current Status Worldwide." *European Journal of Clinical Nutrition.* doi:10.1038/s41430-020-0558-y.

[52] Filipov, J. J., Metodieva, T., Petrova, M., Zlatkov, B. K., and Dimitrov, E. P. 2017. "Treatment of Persistent Secondary Hyperparathyroidism in Hypercalcemic Kidney Transplant Recipients with Cinacalcet: A Single Centre Experience." *Comptes Rendus de L'Academie Bulgare Des Sciences* 70 (11).

[53] Evenepoel, P., Cooper, K., Holdaas, H., Messa, P., Mourad, G., Olgaard, K., Rutkowski, B., Schaefer, H., Deng, H., Torregrosa, J. V., Wuthrich, R. P. and Yue, S. 2014. "A Randomized Study Evaluating Cinacalcet to Treat Hypercalcemia in Renal Transplant

Recipients with Persistent Hyperparathyroidism." *American Journal of Transplantation* 14 (11): 2545–55. doi:10.1111/ajt.12911.

[54] Toth-Manikowski, S M., Francis, J. M., Gautam, A., and Gordon, C. E. 2016. "Outcomes of Bisphosphonate Therapy in Kidney Transplant Recipients: A Systematic Review and Meta-Analysis." *Clinical Transplantation* 30 (9): 1090–96. doi:10.1111/ctr.12792.

[55] Palmer, S. C., Chung, E. Y., McGregor, D. O., Bachmann, F., and Strippoli, G. 2019. "Interventions for Preventing Bone Disease in Kidney Transplant Recipients." *Cochrane Database of Systematic Reviews.* doi: 10.1002/14651858.CD005015.pub4.

[56] Coco, M., Glicklich, D., Faugere, M. C., Burris, L., Bognar, I., Durkin, P., Tellis, V., Greenstein, S., Schechner, R., Figueroa, K., McDonough, P., Wang, G. and Malluche, H. 2003. "Prevention of Bone Loss in Renal Transplant Recipients: A Prospective, Randomized Trial of Intravenous Pamidronate." *Journal of the American Society of Nephrology* 14 (10): 2669–76.

[57] McKee, H., Ioannidis, G., Lau, A., Treleaven, D., Gangji, A., Ribic, C., Wong-Pack, M., Papaioannou, A., and Adachi, J. D. 2020. "Comparison of the Clinical Effectiveness and Safety between the Use of Denosumab vs Bisphosphonates in Renal Transplant Patients." *Osteoporosis International* 31 (5): 973–80. doi:10.1007/s00198-019-05267-1.

[58] Kobel, C., Frey, D., Graf, N., Wüthrich, R. P., and Bonani, M. 2019. "Follow-Up of Bone Mineral Density Changes in de Novo Kidney Transplant Recipients Treated with Two Doses of the Receptor Activator of Nuclear Factor κB Ligand Inhibitor Denosumab." *Kidney and Blood Pressure Research* 44 (5): 1285–93. doi:10.1159/000503066.

[59] Cejka, D., Benesch, T., Krestan, C., Roschger, P., Klaushofer, K., Pietschmann, P., and Haas, M. 2008. "Effect of Teriparatide on Early Bone Loss after Kidney Transplantation." *American Journal of Transplantation* 8 (9): 1864–70. doi:10.1111/j.1600-6143.2008.02327.x.

[60] Cruzado, J. M., Moreno, P., Torregrosa, J. V., Taco, O., Mast, R., Gómez-Vaquero, C., Polo, C., Revuelta, I., Francos, J., Torras, J., García-Barrasa, A., Bestard, O. and Grinyó, Josep M. 2016. "A Randomized Study Comparing Parathyroidectomy with Cinacalcet for Treating Hypercalcemia in Kidney Allograft Recipients with Hyperparathyroidism." *Journal of the American Society of Nephrology* 27 (8): 2487–94. doi:10.1681/ASN.2015060622.

[61] Moreno, P., Coloma, A., Torregrosa, J. V., Montero, N., Francos, J., Codina, S., Manonelles, A., Bestard, O., Garcia-Barrasa, A., Milleli, E. and Cruzado, J. M. 2020. "Long-Term Results of a Randomized Study Comparing Parathyroidectomy with Cinacalcet for Treating Tertiary Hyperparathyroidism." *Clinical Transplantation* 34 (8). doi:10.1111/ctr.13988.

[62] Evenepoel, P., Cunningham, J., Ferrari, S., Haarhaus, M., Javaid, M., Lafage-Proust, M., Prieto-Alhambra, D., Torres, P. U. and Cannata-Andia, Jorge. 2020. "European Consensus Statement on the Diagnosis and Management of Osteoporosis in Chronic Kidney Disease Stages G4–G5D." *Nephrology Dialysis Transplantation*. doi:10.1093/ndt/gfaa192.

[63] Siddique, N., O'Donoghue, M., Casey, M. C., and Walsh, J. B. 2017. "Malnutrition in the Elderly and Its Effects on Bone Health – A Review." *Clinical Nutrition ESPEN* 21: 31–39. doi:10.1016/j.clnesp.2017.06.001.

[64] Kahwaji, J., Bunnapradist, S., Hsu, J. W., Idroos, M. L., and Dudek, R. 2011. "Cause of Death with Graft Function among Renal Transplant Recipients in an Integrated Healthcare System." *Transplantation* 91 (2): 225–30. doi:10.1097/TP.0b013e3181ff8754.

[65] Cianciolo, G., Capelli, I., Angelini, M. L., Valentini, C., Baraldi, O., Scolari, M. P., and Stefoni, S. 2014. "Importance of Vascular Calcification in Kidney Transplant Recipients." *American Journal of Nephrology* 39 (5): 418–26. doi:10.1159/000362492.

[66] Alfieri, C., Forzenigo, L., Tripodi, F., Meneghini, M., Regalia, A., Cresseri, D., and Messa, P. 2019. "Long-Term Evaluation of Coronary Artery Calcifications in Kidney Transplanted Patients: A

Follow up of 5 Years." *Scientific Reports* 9 (1). doi:10.1038/s41598-019-43216-4.

[67] Alappan, H. R., Vasanth, P., Manzoor, S., and O'Neill, W. C. 2020. "Vascular Calcification Slows but Does Not Regress After Kidney Transplantation." *Kidney International Reports*. doi:10.1016/j.ekir.2020.09.039.

[68] Okamoto, M., Yamanaka, S., Yoshimoto, W., and Shigematsu, T. 2014. "Alendronate as an Effective Treatment for Bone Loss and Vascular Calcification in Kidney Transplant Recipients." *Journal of Transplantation* 2014: 1–6. doi:10.1155/2014/269613.

[69] Haugsgjerd, T. R., Egeland, G. M., Nygård, O. K., Vinknes, K. J., Sulo, G., Lysne, V., Igland, J., and Tell, G. S. 2020. "Association of Dietary Vitamin K and Risk of Coronary Heart Disease in Middle-Age Adults: The Hordaland Health Study Cohort." *BMJ Open* 10 (5). doi:10.1136/bmjopen-2019-035953.

[70] Fusaro, M., Plebani, M., Iervasi, G., and Gallieni, M. 2017. "Vitamin K Deficiency in Chronic Kidney Disease: Evidence Is Building Up." *American Journal of Nephrology*. doi:10.1159/000451070.

[71] Raggi, P., Bellasi, A., Bushinsky, D., Bover, J., Rodriguez, M., Ketteler, M., Sinha, S., Salcedo, C., Gillotti, K., Padgett, C., Garg, R., Gold, A., Perelló, J., Chertow, Glenn M. 2020. "Slowing Progression of Cardiovascular Calcification with snf472 in Patients on Hemodialysis: Results of a Randomized Phase 2b Study." *Circulation*, 728–39. doi:10.1161/CIRCULATIONAHA.119.044195.

[72] Zoccali, C., and London, G. 2015. "Con: Vascular Calcification Is a Surrogate Marker, but Not the Cause of Ongoing Vascular Disease, and It Is Not a Treatment Target in Chronic Kidney Disease." *Nephrology Dialysis Transplantation*. doi:10.1093/ndt/gfv021.

In: Kidney Transplantation
Editor: Robert C. Morgan

ISBN: 978-1-53619-721-1
© 2021 Nova Science Publishers, Inc.

Chapter 2

PSYCHOSOCIAL ASSESSMENT OF THE LIVE KIDNEY DONOR AND RECIPIENT

Yasemin Kocyigit[1,],*
Sanem Cimen[2]
and Ayse Gokcen Gundogmus[1]

[1]Department of Psychiatry, University of Health Sciences, Ankara Diskapi Yildirim Beyazit Research and Training Hospital, Ankara, Turkey
[2]Department of Surgery, University of Health Sciences, Ankara Diskapi Yildirim Beyazit Research and Training Hospital, Ankara, Turkey

ABSTRACT

Chronic diseases provoke various psychological and behavioral problems and thus necessitate psychiatric evaluation. One of the most common chronic diseases worldwide is chronic kidney disease. The best treatment method for chronic kidney disease is a live donor kidney transplantation. However, it requires a healthy person, the donor, to undergo a surgical procedure for the sake of a loved one. Unfortunately,

---

[*] Corresponding Author's E-mail: drysmnkcygt@hotmail.com.

after the transplant procedure, poor outcomes related to non-compliance can be recorded in varying ratios. Treatment non-compliance may lead to chronic allograft rejection and loss of the donated kidney. In many cases, an in-depth psychological evaluation can predict adverse post-transplant events such as non-compliance and propose improvement strategies. Therefore, the inclusion of a psychiatrist in the transplant team helps to prevent these undesirable outcomes. When the recipient, living donor, along with their family decides to proceed with the transplant, it is a lifelong commitment. A favorable psychiatric evaluation for both the donor and recipient is a testimony of all participants` willingness and commitment to the best outcome. This review highlights common issues faced at different stages of this lengthy pathway.

Keywords: kidney transplantation, psychological evaluation, psychopathology, live donor

1. INTRODUCTION

The prevalence of chronic diseases such as hypertension and diabetes is increasing. With this increase, the demand for organ transplantation also increases, and despite the technological developments in organ transplantation, problems affecting the success of transplants continue (Black et al., 2018). Scarcity of suitable organs for transplantation, single dimensioned focus on the surgical/medical aspects of the transplant process, and neglecting the mental dimension is a limiting factor to success (De Pasqaule et al., 2020). Careful evaluation of recipient candidates is imperative before listing for a kidney transplant (United Network of Organ Sharing and Scientific Registry of Transplant Recipients, 2019).

The transplant waitlist committee should decide on the transplant recipient list using medical and psychosocial criteria detailed in clinical guidelines (López-Lazcano et al., 2019). The committee should consider the risk factors and medical or psychosocial problems that may prevent a candidate from being placed on the waiting list (Fidel Kinori et al., 2015; Lopez-Lazcano et al., 2019). However, the lack of standardization in psychosocial criteria for all organ and cell transplants can create prejudice and increase ethical concerns in the process of transplant candidate selection (Lewandowski & Skillings, 2016).

Kidney transplantation carries medical risks for the patient and living donor and requires an adaptation process. For this reason, it is necessary to evaluate the recipient and donor candidate's medical and psychosocial aspects before the transplant (Mjøen et al., 2014; Jesse et al., 2019). In the pre-transplant period, the recipient's comprehension of treatment and compliance assessment is paramount. On the donor side, psychological suitability and motivation assessment should be in the foreground. In the post-transplantation period, early detection of psychological problems, treatment planning, and being alert about the side effects and interaction risks of the drugs used constitutes the mainstream (Medved, Medved & Skočić Hanžek, 2019).

1.1. Psychosocial Evaluation of the Recipient in the Pre-Transplant Period

The psychosocial evaluation of the recipient during the pre-transplant period focuses on the suitability of the patient for transplantation, level of mental preparedness, presence of psychological support systems, and covers topics such as functionality, psychological state, and psychopathologies. Mental preparedness comes with knowledge and understanding of the medical disease and the transplantation process, treatment desire, treatment compliance, and lifestyle characteristics such as diet, exercise. Psychopathological assessment should entail many dimensions such as psychopathologic diagnoses, neurocognitive disorders, personality disorders-characteristics, and alcohol-substance abuse (Medved, Medved & Skočić Hanžek, 2019). Psychiatric evaluation in the pre-transplant period is a valuable tool to predict compliance in the post-transplant treatment (Medved, Medved & Skočić Hanžek, 2019; Dew et al., 2000). The association of adverse psychosocial factors with reduced post-transplant survival and high infection rates has been established (Owen, Bonds & Wellisch, 2006). Individuals who underwent kidney transplantation and were evaluated as non-compliant before the procedure had graft loss or death at a rate of 61% in a 3-year follow-up study (Douglas, Blixen & Bartucci, 1996).

Transplantation is a challenging, tiring, and stressful event that requires the patient to use biopsychosocial skills to accept and adapt to a new organ physically and mentally. Emotional and social changes occur in both the patient's and her family's lives, and it requires a certain level of patient readiness for this process to be successful (De Pasquale et al., 2020).

A thorough psychological assessment can identify methods to improve a patient's long-term therapeutic adherence. Long-term compliance is a principal indicator of treatment success. The term compliance not only involves taking medications as prescribed. It also involves changes in life style like being on time for regular check-ups, eating a balanced diet, and exercising daily, and is influenced by many factors such as age, gender, ethnicity, social support, and perceived self-efficacy (Dew et al., 2007a). Noncompliance is related to the complexity of medical prescriptions, personality, life style before transplantation, and patient's clinical features, like long-term dialysis, dementia.

The integrated multidisciplinary assessment and care aim to improve patient's adaptation to surgery, medical treatment, and a healthier lifestyle, developing new coping skills and increasing autonomy (De Pasquale et al., 2014). The psychiatrist's involvement is valuable in understanding the patients` psychological reactions, some of which can otherwise be perceived as non-adherence or early symptoms of a psychiatric disorder by the transplant team. Misunderstandings in communication and misinterpretation of expectations between parties can make the transplantation process difficult.

1.1.1. Assessments

Worldwide, there are different protocols for the psychological evaluation of patients in the transplant process, and there is no specific standardization in this regard, and variations are present among transplant centers. Some centers start patient assessment with screening questionnaires such as general health surveys (Medved, Medved & Skočić Hanžek, 2019). However, the first evaluation is usually the psychiatric evaluation; an unstructured psychiatric clinical interview focusing specifically on risk factors that may impair compliance (Owen, Bonds & Wellisch, 2006; Dwen et al., 2007a; Maldonado, 2019). The unstructured psychiatric interview includes mental state examination, treatment of detected mental illnesses, evaluation of the individual in terms of substance abuse, psychosocial risks, cognitive status, history of educational level and professional life, social support, and medical compliance (Olbrisch et al., 2002).

Following an unstructured interview, the psychiatrist involved in the transplantation process can conduct additional neuropsychological tests and social work evaluations. Diagnosing and treating psychosocial or psychiatric problems in the pre-transplant period improves patient outcomes post-transplant (Dew et al., 2007a).

The 2020 Kidney Disease Improving Global Outcomes (KDIGO) Clinical Practice Guideline addresses issues such as access to transplantation, demographic and health components, immunological and psychosocial assessment of potential recipients (Chadban et al., 2020).

Pre-transplant psychosocial assessment can be classified under some headings (Maldonado, 2009) and should include the following to optimize results and fair and appropriate use of limited resources;

1. Mental state examination to address current psychiatric problems and help minimize psychosocial difficulties, to determine neuropsychiatric state and cognitive functioning skills.
   - Assessment of current and past mental illness (treatment process, remission)
   - History of psychiatric treatments
   - Determining how a psychiatric disorder affects a patient's daily life or decision-making capacity
   - Evaluation of alcohol and substance abuse
   - Assessment of tobacco use history
   - Detection of self-harming thoughts/attempts

- Evaluating the capacity to understand the process and give consent
- Detection of coping styles and personality traits/disorders
- Addressing issues of compliance-competence
2. Patient knowledge regarding treatment options and the severity of side effects
   - Patient awareness on available treatment options
   - Information about the transplantation process (surgery, the short-term and long-term side effects of treatments, possible complications, and risks, required lifestyle changes)
3. Expectations from the outcomes of transplantation
   - Understanding patient's expectations regarding the postoperative period
   - Patient understanding of main medical risks and possible clinical course
   - Expectations for improvement in symptoms and changes in quality of life
   - Awareness of the patient about post-transplant check-ups
4. Evaluation of the support systems to examine the social support network and help strengthen the support systems if there is a deficiency
5. Detection of other problems related to patient and support systems, and obtain the necessary information to develop and implement treatment plans that address psychosocial vulnerabilities for individuals at high risk

1.1.2. Approach to Psychological Conditions and Psychopathologies

The impact of chronic illness and disability expands beyond the individual to everyone they come into contact with, affecting many aspects of life, such as social relationships, family relations, economic well-being, daily activities, leisure, and professional activities. The psychological reaction to the illness depend on many factors such as the nature of the illness, the personality traits, and the maturation of the patient. This reaction can include offense, depression, a desire to be isolated, and is not necessarily pathological. Clinical depression should be differentiated from burnout related to chronic diseases. Psychological burnout can manifest itself as a lack of willpower, fatigue, and attention deficit and is a reaction observed while hustling with a chronic illness (Medved, Medved & Skočić Hanžek, 2019).

Psychological reactions may be more intense in terminally ill patients awaiting transplantation (Medved, Medved & Skočić Hanžek, 2019). Although entering the transplant list is seen as a chance for a new life by the patient and is greeted with enthusiasm, long waiting periods with little contact with the transport team may cause patients to feel anger and abandonment (Hoffman, Saulino & Smith, 2019). Thus, several studies on transplant-waitlisted patients found that the most common psychological problem in patients awaiting kidney transplantation was noncompliance, as well as depression, anxiety, and adjustment disorders (Naqvi, 2015; Rogal et al., 2011). An approximately 20-30% of hemodialysis patients present symptoms consistent with major depressive disorder (Zalai, Szeifert & Novak, 2012; Avramovic & Stefanovic, 2012). In patients with chronic renal failure depression, disrupts medical treatment compliance (DiMatteo, Lepper & Croghan, 2000), decreases the quality of life, increases the risk of graft loss and mortality after transplant (Zalai, Szeifert & Novak, 2012; Corruble et al., 2011; Cukor et al., 2009). On the other hand, few studies show that depressive symptoms in the pre-transplant period may not be directly related to negative clinical results (Corruble et al., 2011). It has been shown that there is a relationship between psychosocial vulnerability before transplantation and adverse outcomes such as infection, noncompliance, re-hospitalization, increased cost of care, post-transplant malignancy, and reduced transplant survival (Maldonado, 2019). In a study conducted on individuals diagnosed with bipolar and psychotic disorders among the patient groups with the above risk factors, disease relapse, recurrent hospitalizations, and poor therapeutic adhesion were found in approximately half of the patients after organ transplantation in their 5-year follow-up (Kofman et al., 2018).

Another group of mental illness is personality disorders. Personality disorders involve long-term patterns of thoughts and behaviors that are unhealthy and inflexible. Thus, personality is one of the aspects to be considered in transplant evaluation (Telles-Correia, Barbosa & Mega,

2010; Zhang et al., 2005; Naqvi, 2015). It can be a risk factor for poor outcomes in the post-transplant period (Dobbels, Put & Vanhaecke, 2000). Among personality disorders, especially neuroticism has been associated with lower quality of life after transplantation (Thomas, de Castro & Antonello, 2016; Prihodova et al., 2009).

1.1.3. Cognitive Assessment

One of the eminent dimensions of psychiatric evaluation in the pre-transplant period is assessing patients' ability to give informed consent. There are three main elements to figure the ability to provide informed consent. These elements are the knowledge about the transplantation process, the ability to understand and make independent decisions.

After the individual is informed by the transplant surgeon about the transplantation process, the severity of the disease leading to organ failure, the meaning of the transplant procedure, the possible problems and complications, the patient's understanding of the process should be evaluated by the psychiatrist for informed consent (Ilić and Avramović, 2002). It should be kept in mind that each patient will perceive the information provided differently, and this perception will be affected by factors such as age, marital status and education level (Ahsanuddin et al., 2015). Besides, since the waiting period between enrollment in the transplant list and transplant may take several years, psychiatric evaluations should be repeated when necessary. Repetition of information and patient-tailored training is required in patients with chronic renal failure with cognitive impairments (Cambell et al., 2012).

1.1.4. Social Support Assessment

Social support is not closely associated with post-transplant outcomes. Post-transplant outcomes were closely associated with return to work, presence of disability, and participation in leisure time activities (Ladin et al., 2018; Weng et al., 2014). Therefore, substantial prospective studies are needed to justify lack of social support as a contraindication for transplantation (Ladin et al., 2018).In general, it is acknowledged that a stable and strong social support is considered as an important denominator for transplant success. Although some guidelines do not focus on this issue, there are some who emphasize the importance of social support, especially in patients with cognitive or neuropsychiatric deficits.

1.1.5. Assessment Tools

Although there is no standardized method for evaluating recipient candidates, transplant centers worldwide are utilizing miscellaneous tools. The validity and reliability studies of these tools are present for various languages. Below, listed some of the widely used tools for assessment purposes (Maldonado, 2019):

1. The Psychosocial Assessment of Candidates for Transplantation (PACT) (Olbrisch, Levenson & Hamer,1989)
2. The Psychosocial Levels System (PLS) (Futterman et al., 1991).
3. The Transplant Evaluation Rating Scale (TERS), a revision of the PLS, (Twillman et al., 1993).
4. the Structured Interview for Renal Transplantation (SIRT) (Mori, Gallagher & Milne, 2000)
5. 2012-SIPAT Stanford Integrated Psychosocial Assessment for Transplantation (Maldonado et al., 2012)
6. mPACT Modified PACT, Revision of PACT for VAD patients, (Maltby et al., 2014)
7. SIPAT-MCS (2018) Stanford Integrated Psychosocial Assessment for Transplantation – Cardiac Mechanical Circulatory Support (MCS) Version-Adaptation of the SIPAT MCS) (Maldonado, 2019).

It is imperative to remember that these tools can aid in the assessment, but they will not be sufficient alone to evaluate candidacy for transplantation (Chadban et al., 2020). SIPAT, one of the evaluation tools listed above, is used more frequently and takes 18 defined risk factors into account in 4 main areas such as patient readiness level and illness management, social support system, psychologic stability and present psychopathologies, as well as substance abuse.

1.1.6. Psychosocial Requirements for Renal Transplantation

There are no national standards or minimum psychosocial requirements to appraise the renal transplant recipient (Maldonado, 2019; Chadban et al., 2020). Although there is a wide array of differences between studies and centers, the criteria listed in Table 1 could help clinicians to determine absolute and relative risk factors in clinical practice. Despite this, we recommend transplant teams to analyze relative contraindications, and absolute contraindications on a case-by-case basis.

Table 1. Relative and Absolute Psychological Contraindications for Recipients

Relative Contraindications	Absolute Contraindications*
• Noncompliance • Presence of a mental illness under clinical follow-up with moderate symptoms (depression, anxiety disorder, obsessive-compulsive disorder, psychotic disorder, mental retardation) • Lack of motivation for the transplantation process • Limited family and social support • Personality disorders • Ongoing alcohol abuse • Ambivalence or denial related to the need for transplantation • Deceptive behaviors • Suicidal thoughts (without any past attempts) • Cognitive disorders	• Acute and severe psychiatric illnesses that reduce the patient's functionality and compromise treatment compliance • Medium-severe mental retardation • Severe dementia • Personality disorders with advanced behavioral and adjustment problems • Alcohol-substance abuse (frequent relapses without treatment) • Ongoing alcohol-substance abuse disorder despite high medical risk • Suicidal thoughts (with past attempts)

*Should be evaluated on a case-by-case basis.

In agreement with this, some guidelines do not qualify a few of the psychiatric illnesses and symptoms listed in the table as contraindications or obstacles (Chadban et al., 2020; Dew et al., 2000; Medved, Medved & Skočić Hanžek, 2019). According to the KDIGO guideline updated in 2020, individuals with an unstable psychiatric disorder and ongoing substance abuse that impair decision-making ability and generate risk after transplant should be considered unsuitable for transplantation. On the other hand, the same guideline recommends individuals without social support but with high self-care capacities and support plans be waitlisted. It also advocates that non-progressive intellectual, cognitive or developmental disabilities should not prevent an individual from receiving a transplant.

There is an increased prevalence of psychiatric presentations in transplant patients; thus, having a psychiatrist with their unique vantage point should be a routine for transplant teams. The decision on the suitability of the individual for transplantation should be made jointly by the treatment team after the evaluation of the psychiatrist, considering the effect of the severity of the current psychiatric situation on the patient's decision-making capacity, adaptation and readiness.

1.2. Psychosocial Evaluation of the Live Donor

Donation from living donors is increasing. Living donor kidney donation provides numerous advantages to the recipient. Firstly, live donor organs are in good condition, as donors go through a tedious selection process beforehand to ensure their kidney function, compatibility, and overall physical/mental health meet the criteria. Secondly, kidneys from living donors function immediately, setting up the recipient for the best short- and long-term outcomes. Lastly, a live donor kidney transplant is scheduled in advance. Thus, it gives the recipient and donor a chance to increase their preparedness level (Hoffman, Saulino & Smith, 2019). Also, a small proportion of donors may experience negative psychosocial effects, such as fatigue, anxiety, depression, health, and financial adverse effects (Hoffman, Saulino & Smith, 2019; Schover et al., 1997; Clemens et al., 2006). On the other hand, improved self-esteem and interpersonal communication with the recipient are also frequently observed (Dew et al., 2007b, Duerinckx et al., 2014).

The donor evaluation should be performed by an experienced psychiatrist, and at least part of this interview should be one on one to free the donor of potential stressors (Hoffman, Saulino & Smith, 2019). Psychosocial evaluation should be done in two stages, first, an initial screening, and second, extensive psychosocial evaluation. It's been recommended these assessments to come before invasive and expensive medical tests (Duerinckx et al., 2014). Psychiatrists need to understand the donor's knowledge of the transplant process and whether the decision to donate is voluntary (Medved, Medved & Skočić Hanžek, 2019). A distinct subgroup of donors is the non-directed donor (NDD) or altruistic donor who decides to donate an organ to a stranger. However, these good-willed individuals were inclined to change their minds when informed about the donation process (Sawinski & Locke, 2019).

Table 2. Potential risk factors to be considered in donor evaluation

High Risk Donor	Low Risk Donor
Psychiatric disease impairing decision making	No previous and current psychiatric disease
Alcohol or substance abuse	No substance abuse
Inadequate economic capability	Financial stability
Reduced ability to comprehend donor risks	Demonstrating good comprehension skills
Ambivalence about donation	Realistic expectations related to donation
Financially motivated	Altruistically motivated
Unreasonable adaptation to life stressors	Examples of resilience to stressors in the past
Subordinate relationship with the recipient	No evidence of coercion
Family not supporting donation	Knowledge and approval by family
Poor family relationships	Strong and healthy family relationships

The decision to donate can be an impulsive one triggered by financial expectations or family pressure. If the donor is a family member of the recipient; the strength of family ties, the number of family members, the relation of the donor to recipient, and the distribution of power within the family, in short, family dynamics is a crucial denominator. Kidney recipients who end up with a failed graft may develop feelings of guilt towards the donor and family. They may also be afraid of asking for further support like another live donor. In this case, the psychiatrist should provide psychological support and counseling to the patient to understand and relieve emotional tension and other possible psychological reactions (Medved, Medved & Skočić Hanžek, 2019).

It is necessary to protect the donor from medical and psychosocial harm. Risk factors associated with negative psychological consequences for the donor are; financial motivation, feeling compelled to donate, concerns about the health effects of donating, high levels of ambivalence, presence of psychiatric illness, presence of unfavorable family relationships, being single, and financial difficulties (Table 2) (Shenoy, 2019; Keven & Aktürk, 2016; Duerinckx et al., 2014).

After the donor organ donation is approved by the transplant team, it is a good practice to give the donor a week to contemplate (Duerinckx et al., 2014). Additionally, meeting with an independent living donor advocate, not involved in the recipient's care, can aid in the articulation of concerns and questions by the donor. This advocate should emphasize the right to withdraw from donation at all times and ensure the safety of the donor (Shenoy, 2019). Informed consent is the ethical bedrock fundamental to living organ donation. Thus, it should be tailored to involve the surgical technique and include a comprehensive description of the risks associated with the donation (Hoffman, Saulino & Smith, 2019).

The psychiatric evaluation of donors should begin with an assessment of autonomy (ability to decide freely, without being under pressure/coercion) and competence (having the cognitive competence and mental health required to make decisions) (Noyan et al., 2011). Assessment of donors includes the following topics and objectives:

1. Mental state examination
   - Obtaining a comprehensive cross-section of the current state of mind with a combination of psychiatric history
   - Evaluation of alcohol-substance abuse
   - Assessment of self-mutilative behavior
   - Identifying suicide ideation and suicidal attempts
   - Examining decision-making capacity and consent processes

- Appraisal of personality traits and coping styles
2. Evaluating the motivation
    - Evaluating the altruism and the desire to benefit someone other than oneself
    - Scrutinizing for the presence of influence exertion by others, feelings of being under pressure, such as demands, threats, or personal attacks from other people
    - Examining potential financial expectations with the donation and the nature of the relationship with the recipient
    - Investigating the effects of factors such as guilt and impulsivity in the decision of donation
    - Inspecting the presence of ambivalence regarding donation
    - Making sure that the donor id aware of alternative treatment options for the recipient
3. Examining donor's knowledge on potential outcomes
    - Understanding the donors` comprehension related to the risks and possible medical course
    - Checking the awareness regarding the possibility of rejection and primary non-function
    - Understanding the donor's expectations after the surgery (relations with the recipient, long-term well-being, return to previous functionality, etc.)
    - Assessing the awareness related to effects of donation in different aspects of life (such as work, insurance)
4. Evaluation of the support system
5. Reviewing the readiness for medical, emotional, and financial effects of donation
    - Ability to anticipate possible difficulties after donation
    - Awareness of post-donation risk factors such as diabetes or hypertension
6. Appraising the knowledge regarding post-donation requirements
    - Awareness of post-donation follow-up visits
    - Presence of health insurance

7. Other: Addressing other questions/concerns of the donor and support system

As a result of the extensive evaluation process, the donor candidate can be found appropriate or not. Rarely, some conditions are recommended to be changed or modified to proceed with the donation process.

The following can be used as psychosocial assessment tools in the evaluation of donors,

1. The Living Donation Expectancies Questionnaire (LDEQ) (Rodrigue et al., 2008)
2. The Rotterdam Renal Replacement Knowledge-Test (R3K-T) for kidney donors (Ismail et al., 2013)
3. The Evaluation of Donor Informed Consent Tool (EDICT) for liver donors (Gordon et al., 2015)
4. The Donation Cognition Instrument (DCI) (Wirken et al., 2017)
5. Live Donor Assessment Tool (LDAT) (Iacoviello et al., 2017)
6. The living organ donor Psychosocial Assessment Tool (EPAT) (Massey et al., 2018)

Comprehensive evaluation of donors is essential to predict ones that may have a negative donation experience. However, there is no standardized approach to the psychosocial evaluation. There is also no validated psychometric tool to determine psychosocial risks for donation.For the validity of the assessment tools listed above, further research is warranted.

1.3. Post-Transplant Follow-Up

Patients with chronic kidney failure who have undergone kidney transplantation have a longer lifespan than dialysis patients. Besides, their quality of life and functionality is better (Joshi, Almeida & Almeida, 2013). Therefore, post-transplant follow-up is paramount to ensure long-term graft and patient survival. In these follow-ups, the progress of recipients should be examined by the transplant nephrologist and surgeon, as well as psychologists and social workers (Keven & Aktürk, 2016).

Considering the altering psychological conditions of kidney recipients, a psychiatrist should also be included in the follow-up. A psychiatrist can recognize the psychological stages the recipient goes through and recommend adjustments. The stages recipient goes through do not follow an order but usually begin with the honeymoon stage. For many patients, this stage starts right after the transplantation. It is a consequence of relief from the restrictions of life on dialysis. Feelings of happiness and well-being predominate the mood during this stage (De Pasquale et al., 2014; Surman, 1989). The duration of the honeymoon stage differs widely. After the honeymoon stage, the recipient may develop fears, such as fear of infection, fear of losing the graft (De Pasquale et al., 2014; Schulz & Kroencke, 2015; Ilić & Avramović, 2002; Surman, 1989). Also, feelings of guilt towards the donor may be observed. Rarely, the recipient may deem transplant as a threat to identity continuity or a violation of personal integrity. In such rare cases, the transplant process can become a traumatic rather than a positive experience (De Pasquale et al., 2014). Transplant experience may also cause post-traumatic growth (psychological maturation) in a small number of patients. This maturation manifests itself as feeling stronger or more creative, as well as increased sociability, and patients feel grateful to have a second chance in life (Zoellner & Maercker, 2006).

On the other hand, compliance and adaptation problems after transplant may torment the recipient in the postoperative course. For example, noncompliance to immunosuppressive treatment leads to complications and even graft failure (Maldonado, 2019). Thus, it is essential to supervene recipient compliance. Factors such as age, gender, self-efficacy level, lifestyle, personality traits (irritable, depressive temperament, cyclothymic) were found to be associated with treatment noncompliance (Denhaerynck et al., 2007; De Pasquale et al., 2014). Other risk factors for noncompliance can be listed as; inadequate pre-transplant education, adolescence, presence of drug side effects, insufficient social support, high education level, complex treatment protocols, incompatibility in previous transplantation, not being followed by the primary transplant physician, presence of psychiatric illness, substance abuse (Keven & Aktürk, 2016). Self-efficacy is associated with improved adherence in kidney transplant recipients. It is inversely related to depressive symptoms (Paterson et al., 2018). The literature emphasizes the significance of present psychopathologies such as anxiety, depression, cognitive disorders, and sleep disorders, which may impair treatment compliance (De Pasquale et al., 2020). There are also studies showing that the relation of perceived stress and depression with treatment noncompliance disappears after controlling for sociodemographic factors (Weng et al., 2013). Cognitive function improvement can be seen after transplantation, and studies (Griva et al., 2004) indicate that patients with an awareness of cognitive dysfunction show greater compliance with immunosuppressant drugs (Cheng et al., 2012).

It is recommended to support transplanted recipients for self-efficacy and resilience to help them adapt to the post-transplant processes (De Pasquale et al., 2020). The recipient and the family-support system must cooperate with the transplant team at all times, especially about the required lifestyle changes, such as healthy diet and exercise (Raiesifar et al., 2014; Zhu et al., 2017). Returning to work, especially after transplantation, is one of the important indicators of psychosocial well-being (De Pasquale et al., 2019; Pistorio et al., 2013 Ahsanuddin et al., 2015). Therefore, attention should be paid to this area in post-transplant follow-ups.

Post-transplant psychiatric complications due to the use of steroids and immunosuppressive drugs are not uncommon and the patient should be warned of the possible physical and mental effects of these drugs. Depressive symptoms, restlessness, euphoria, confusion, and paranoid reactions (Steroid psychosis) with hallucinations can be seen due to steroid use (Ilić & Avramović, 2002).

When complications occur in the post-transplant course, they may cause feelings of guilt and anger in donors and may trigger depression (Parikh et al., 2010). Donors can also experience psychosocial difficulties after the transplant, similar to recipients, such as depression (5-23%), anxiety (6-14%), stress (6-22%), health concerns (6-50%) (Clemens et al., 2006). It has been reported that guilt (5%) and suicidal thoughts (11%) have been observed in donors (Clemens et al., 2006). Therefore, donors should also be followed-up psychologically in the post-transplant period.

CONCLUSION

Although kidney transplant is a life-saving treatment option, it brings many psychological, social, legal, and ethical problems. Considering the important psychosocial problems that can be encountered at all stages of the transplantation process, psychiatrists are needed as a member of the multidisciplinary team (Ilić and Avramović, 2002). Psychiatric consultation before transplant is aimed at evaluating the psychosocial suitability of the transplant, cognitive state, and decision-making capacity. The assessment is carried out through mental state examination, psychosocial status assessment, and, when necessary, psychometric and cognitive tests. Psychiatrists should consider the risk of exacerbation or recurrence of the previous diseases in individuals with mental illnesses. The psychiatrist's assessment of the patient's psychosocial suitability ends with an overview of their strengths and possible limitations and provides a summary of the interventions proposed to optimize the patient's transplant candidacy. It is known from both clinical practice and scientific data that psychiatric consultation has an important role in the comprehensive selection of candidates. In the donation process, psychiatrists should evaluate the donor's psychological suitability and motivation, especially the donor's autonomy and competence. In the post-transplant period, the follow-up of the psychological state of the individuals and their compliance with the treatment process is important for the management and success of the process. Another task of psychiatrists is to organize the relationship between the transplant team and the patient when necessary and to help the medical team to see each patient as an individual with a special and different set of needs and expectations (Medved, Medved &

Skočić Hanžek, 2019). Psychiatric interventions do not only meet the needs of transplant candidates. It also plays a role in effective use of limited resources and increasing social functionality due to transplant procedures (Medved, Medved & Skočić Hanžek, 2019).

REFERENCES

Ahsanuddin, Sayeeda, Sandra Bento, Nicholas Swerdlow, Ixel Cervera, and Liise K. Kayler. 2015. "Candidate Comprehension of Key Concepts in Kidney Transplantation." *Annals of Transplantation: Quarterly of the Polish Transplantation Society* 20: 124–31.

Avramovic, Marina and Vladisav Stefanovic. 2012. "Health-Related Quality of Life in Different Stages of Renal Failure." *Artificial organs*, 36(7), 581-589.

Black, Cara K., Kareem M. Termanini, Oswaldo Aguirre, Jason S. Hawksworth, and Michael Sosin. 2018. "Solid Organ Transplantation in the 21st Century." *Annals of Translational Medicine* 6 (20): 409–409.

Campbell, Noll L., Malaz A. Boustani, Elaine N. Skopelja, Sujuan Gao, Fred W. Unverzagt, Michael D. Murray 2012. "Medication Adherence in Older Adults with Cognitive Impairment: A Systematic Evidence-Based Review." *Am J Geriatr Pharmacother*; 10:165e77. Https://Doi. Org/10, 04 004.

Chadban, Steven J., Curie Ahn, David A. Axelrod, Bethany J. Foster, Bertram L. Kasiske, Vijah Kher, Deepali Kumar, et al. 2020. "KDIGO Clinical Practice Guideline on the Evaluation and Management of Candidates for Kidney Transplantation." *Transplantation* 104 (4S1): S11–103.

Clemens, Kristen K., Heather Thiessen-Philbrook, Chirag. R. Parikh, R. C. Yang, M. L. Karley, Neil Boudville, G. V. Ramesh Prasad, A. X. Garg, and Donor Nephrectomy Outcomes Research (DONOR) Network. 2006. "Psychosocial Health of Living Kidney Donors: A Systematic Review." *American Journal of Transplantation: Official Journal of the*

American Society of Transplantation and the American Society of Transplant Surgeons 6 (12): 2965–77.

Corruble, Emmanuelle, Caroline Barry, Isabelle Varescon, Antoine Durrbach, Didier Samuel, Philippe Lang, Denis Castaing, Bernard Charpentier, and Bruno Falissard. 2011. "Report of Depressive Symptoms on Waiting List and Mortality after Liver and Kidney Transplantation: A Prospective Cohort Study." *BMC Psychiatry* 11 (1). https://doi.org/10.1186/1471-244x-11-182.

Cukor, Daniel, Deborah S. Rosenthal, Rahul M. Jindal, Clinton D. Brown, and Paul L. Kimmel. 2009. "Depression Is an Important Contributor to Low Medication Adherence in Hemodialyzed Patients and Transplant Recipients." *Kidney International* 75 (11): 1223–29.

Cheng C-Y., B Y-J Lin, K-H Chang, K-H Shu, M-J Wu 2012. "Awareness of Memory Impairment Increases the Adherence To Immunosuppressants In Kidney Transplant Recipients." *Transplant Proc* 44 (746): 11 030.

De Pasquale, Concetta, Maria Luisa Pistorio, Massimiliano Veroux, Luisa Indelicato, Gabriella Biffa, Nunzialinda Bennardi, Pietro Zoncheddu, Valentina Martinelli, Alessia Giaquinta, and Pierfrancesco Veroux. 2020. "Psychological and Psychopathological Aspects of Kidney Transplantation: A Systematic Review." *Frontiers in Psychiatry* 11: 106.

De Pasquale, Concetta, Massimiliano Veroux, Luisa Indelicato, Nunzia Sinagra, Alessia Giaquinta, Michele Fornaro, Pierfrancesco Veroux, and Maria L. Pistorio. 2014. "Psychopathological Aspects of Kidney Transplantation: Efficacy of a Multidisciplinary Team." *World Journal of Transplantation* 4 (4): 267–75.

De Pasquale, Concetta, Massimiliano Veroux, Maria Luisa Pistorio, Agata Papotto, Giuseppe Basile, Marco Patanè, Pierfran-cesco Veroux, Alessia Giaquinta and Federica Sciacca. 2019. "Return to Work and Quality of Life: A Psychosocial Survey after Kidney Transplant." *Transplantation Proceedings* 51 (1): 153–56. https://doi.org/10.1016/j.transproceed.2018.04.083.

Denhaerynck, Kris, J. Steiger, A. Bock, Petra Schäfer-Keller, S. Köfer, N. Thannberger, and Sabina De Geest. 2007. "Prevalence and Risk Factors of Non-Adherence with Immunosuppressive Medication in Kidney Transplant Patients." *American Journal of Transplantation: Official Journal of the American Society of Transplantation and the American Society of Transplant Surgeons* 7 (1): 108–16.

Dew, Mary Amanda, Andrea F. DiMartini, Annette De Vito Dabbs, Larissa Myaskovsky, Jennifer Steel, Mark Unruh, Galen E. Switzer, RachelleZomak, Robert L. Kormos, and Joel B. Greenhouse. 2007. "Rates and Risk Factors for Nonadherence to the Medical Regimen after Adult Solid Organ Transplantation." *Transplantation* 83 (7): 858–73.

Dew, Mary Amanda, Galen Switzer, Andrea DiMartini, Jennifer Matukaitis, Mary Fitzgerald, and Robert Kormos. 2000. "Psychosocial Assessments and Outcomes in Organ Transplantation." *Progress in Transplantation* (Aliso Viejo, Calif.) 10 (4): 239–61.

Dew, Mary Amanda, Galen E. Switzer, Andrea F. Dimartini, Larissa Myaskovsky, and, Megan Crowley-Matoka. 2007. *"Psychoso-cial Aspects of Living Organ Donation."* In edited by H. Tan, A. Marcos, and R. Shapiro. New York: Taylor and Francis, 7–26.

DiMatteo, M. Robin, Heidi S. Lepper, and Thomas W. Croghan. 2000. "Depression Is a Risk Factor for Noncompliance with Medical Treatment: Meta-Analysis of the Effects of Anxiety and Depression on Patient Adherence." *Archives of Internal Medicine* 160 (14): 2101.

Dobbels, Fabienne, Claudia Put, and Johan Vanhaecke. 2000. "Personality Disorders: A Challenge for Transplantation." *Progress in Transplantation* (Aliso Viejo, Calif.) 10 (4): 226–32.

Douglas, Sara, Carol Blixen, and Marilyn Bartucci. 1996. "Relationship between Pretransplant Noncompliance and Posttransplant Outcomes in Renal Transplant Recipients." *Journal of Transplant Coordination: Official Publication of the North American Transplant Coordinators Organization* (NATCO) 6 (2): 53–58.

Duerinckx, Nathalie, Lotte Timmerman, Johan Van Gogh, Jan van Busschbach, Sohal Y. Ismail, Emma K. Massey, Fabienne Dobbels, and ELPAT Psychological Care for Living Donors and Recipients working group. 2014. "Predonation Psychosocial Evaluation of Living Kidney and Liver Donor Candidates: A Systematic Literature Review." *Transplant International: Official Journal of the European Society for Organ Transplantation* 27 (1): 2–18.

Futterman, Ann D., David K. Wellisch, Gayle Bond, and Clifford R. Carr. 1991. "The Psychosocial Levels System." *Psychosomatics* 32 (2): 177–86.

Gordon, Elisa J., Jack Mullee, Zeeshan Butt, Joseph Kang, and Talia Baker. 2015. "Optimizing Informed Consent in Living Liver Donors: Evaluation of a Comprehension Assessment Tool: Informed Consent in Living Liver Donors." *Liver Transplantation: Official Publication of the American Association for the Study of Liver Diseases and the International Liver Transplantation Society* 21 (10): 1270–79.

Griva, Konstadina, Sunita Hansraj, Derek Thompson, Dakshina Jayasena, Andrew Davenport, Michael Harrison, Stanton P Newman 2004. "Neuropsychological Performance after Kidney Transplantation: A Comparison between Transplant Types and in Relation to Dialysis and Normative Data." *Nephrology, Dialysis, Transplantation: Official Publication of the European Dialysis and Transplant Association - European Renal Association* 19 (7): 1866–74.

Hoffman, Benson M., Caroline K. Saulino, and Patrick J. Smith. 2019. "Psychosocial Aspects of Kidney Transplantation and Living Kidney Donation." In *Kidney Transplantation - Principles and Practice*, 709–23. Elsevier.

Iacoviello, Brian M., Akhil Shenoy, Julia Hunt, Zorica Filipovic-Jewell, Brandy Haydel, and Dianne LaPointe Rudow. 2017. "A Prospective Study of the Reliability and Validity of the Live Donor Assessment Tool." *Psychosomatics* 58 (5): 519–26.

Ilić, Slobodan, and Marina Avramović. 2002. "Psychological Aspects Of Living Donor Kidney Transplantation." *Med Biol* 9: 195–200.

Ismail, Sohal Y., Lotte Timmerman, Reinier Timman, Annemarie E. Luchtenburg, Peter J. H. Smak Gregoor, Robert W. Nette, René M. A. van den Dorpel, et al. 2013. "A Psychometric Analysis of the

Rotterdam Renal Replacement Knowledge-Test (R3K-T) Using Item Response Theory." *Transplant International: Official Journal of the European Society for Organ Transplantation* 26 (12): 1164–72.

Jesse, Michelle T., Anne Eshelman, Teresa Christian, Marwan Abouljoud, Jason Denny, Anita Patel, and Dean Y. Kim. 2019. "Psychiatric Profile of Patients Currently Listed for Kidney Transplantation: Evidence of the Need for More Thorough Pretransplant Psychiatric Evaluations." *Transplantation Proceedings* 51 (10): 3227–33.

Joshi S.A., N. Almeida, and Anda Almeida. 2013. "Assessment of the Perceived Quality of Life of Successful Kidney Transplant Recipients and Their Donors Pre- and Post-Transplantation." *Transplant Proc* 45 (1435): 01 037.

Keven, Kenan, Serkan Aktürk. 2016. *Transplantasyona Hazırlık - Verici-Transplantasyon Nefrolojisi Pratik Uygulama Rehberi*, 9-26.Türk Nefroloji Derneği. [*Preparation for Transplantation - Donor - Transplantation of Nephrology Practical Application Guide*, 9-26.Turkish Nephrology Association.]

Kofman, Tomek, Franck Pourcine, Florence Canoui-Poitrine, Nassim Kamar, Paolo Malvezzi, Hélène François, Emmanuelle Boutin, et al. 2018. "Safety of Renal Transplantation in Patients with Bipolar or Psychotic Disorders: A Retrospective Study." *Transplant International: Official Journal of the European Society for Organ Transplantation* 31 (4): 377–85.

Ladin, Keren, Alexis Daniels, Mikala Osani, and Raveendhara R. Bannuru. 2018. "Is Social Support Associated With Post-Transplant Medication Adherence And Outcomes? A Systematic Review and Meta-Analysis." *Transplant Rev,* 04 001.

Lewandowski, Amber N., and Jared Lyon Skillings. 2016. "Who Gets a Lung Transplant? Assessing the Psychosocial Decision-Making Process for Transplant Listing." *Global Cardiology Science & Practice* 2016 (3). https://doi.org/10.21542/gcsp.2016.26.

López-Lazcano, Ana Isabel, Hugo López-Pelayo, Anna Lligoña, Nuria Sánchez, Vanessa Vilas-Riotorto, Angel Priego, Roberto Sánchez-González, et al. 2019. "Translation, Adaptation, and

Reliability of the Stanford Integrated Psychosocial Assessment for Transplantation in the Spanish Population." *Clinical Transplantation* 33 (10). https://doi.org/10.1111/ctr.13688.

Maldonado, José R. 2009. "I Have Been Asked to Work up a Patient Who Requires a Liver Transplant How Should I Proceed?" *Focus* 7 (3).

Maldonado, José R. 2019. "The Psychosocial Evaluation of Transplant Candidates." In *Psychosocial Care of End-Stage Organ Disease and Transplant Patients*, 17–48. Cham: Springer International Publishing.

Maldonado, José R., Holly C. Dubois, Evonne E. David, Yelizaveta Sher, Sermsak Lolak, Jameson Dyal, and Daniela Witten. 2012. "The Stanford Integrated Psychosocial Assessment for Transplantation (SIPAT): A New Tool for the Psychosocial Evaluation of Pre-Transplant Candidates." *Psychosomatics* 53 (2): 123–32.

Maltby, Megan C., Maureen P. Flattery, Brigid Burns, Jeanne Salyer, Stephan Weinland, and Keyur B. Shah. 2014. "Psychosocial Assessment of Candidates and Risk Classification of Patients Considered for Durable Mechanical Circulatory Support." *The Journal of Heart and Lung Transplantation: The Official Publication of the International Society for Heart Transplantation* 33 (8): 836–41.

Massey, Emma K., Lotte Timmerman, Sohal Y. Ismail, Nathalie Duerinckx, Alice Lopes, Hannah Maple, Inês Mega, Christina Papachristou, Fabienne Dobbels, and the ELPAT Psychosocial Care for Living Donors and Recipients Working Group. 2018. "The ELPAT Living Organ Donor Psychosocial Assessment Tool (EPAT): From 'What' to 'How' of Psychosocial Screening - a Pilot Study." *Transplant International: Official Journal of the European Society for Organ Transplantation* 31 (1): 56–70.

Medved, Vesna, Sara Medved, and Milena Skočić Hanžek. 2019. "Transplantation Psychiatry: An Overview." *Psychiatria Danubina* 31 (1): 18–25.

Mjøen, Geir, Stein Hallan, Anders Hartmann, Aksel Foss, KarstenMidtvedt, Ole Øyen, Anna Reisæter, et al. 2014. "Long-Term Risks for Kidney Donors." *Kidney International* 86 (1): 162–67.

Mori, Deanna L., Patricia Gallagher and Judith Milne 2000. "The Structured Interview for Renal Transplantation—SIRT." *Psychosomatics* 41(5):393-406.

Naqvi, Rubina. 2015. "Evaluation of Psychiatric Issues in Renal Transplant Setting." *Indian Journal of Nephrology* 25 (6): 321.

Noyan, Aysın M., Ozen O. Sertoz, Hayriye Elbi, Ozgul Cetin. 2011. "Canlıdan organ naklinde ruhsal değerlendirme" *Anadolu Psikiyatri Dergisi.* ["Psychiatric assessment in living donation." *Anatolian Journal of Psychiatry*]; 12:84-89.

Olbrisch, Mary E., James E. Levenson, and Robert Hamer. 1989. "The Pact: A Rating Scale for The Study of Clinical Decision Making in Psychosocial Screening of Organ Transplant Candidates." *Clin Transpl* 3: 164–9.

Olbrisch, Mary E., Sharon M. Benedict, Kristine Ashe and, James L. Levenson 2002. "Psychological Assessment and Care of Organ Transplant Patients." *J Consult Clin Psychol* Jun; 70(3):771-83. doi: 10: 1037 0022–006.

Owen, Jason E., Curley L. Bonds, and David K. Wellisch. 2006. "Psychiatric Evaluations of Heart Transplant Candidates: Predicting Post-Transplant Hospitalizations, Rejection Episodes, and Survival." *Psychosomatics* 47 (3): 213–22.

Parikh, Neehar D., Daniela Ladner, Michael Abecassis, and Zeeshan Butt. 2010. "Quality of Life for Donors after Living Donor Liver Transplantation: A Review of the Literature." *Liver Transplantation: Official Publication of the American Association for the Study of Liver Diseases and the International Liver Transplantation Society* 16 (12): 1352–58.

Paterson, Theone S. E., Norm O'Rourke, R. Jean Shapiro, and Wendy Loken Thornton. 2018. "Medication Adherence in Renal Transplant Recipients: A Latent Variable Model of Psychosocial and Neurocognitive Predictors." *PloS One* 13 (9): e0204219.

Pistorio, Maria Luisa, Massimiliano Veroux, Daniela Corona, Nunzia Sinagra, Alessia Giaquinta, Domenico Zerbo, Francesco Giacchi, et al. 2013. "The Study of Personality in Renal Transplant Patients: Possible

Predictor of an Adequate Social Adaptation?" *Transplantation Proceedings* 45 (7): 2657–59.

Prihodova, Lucia, Iveta Nagyova, Jaroslav Rosenberger, Robert Roland, Jitse P van Dijk, Johan W Groothoff. 2009. "Impact of Personality and Psychological Distress on Health-Related Quality of Life in Kidney Transplant Recipients." *Transplant International* 23 (5): 484–492.

Raiesifar, Afsaneh, Ali Tayebi, Soheil Najafi Mehrii, Abbas Ebadi, Behzad Einollahi, Hadi Tabibi, Parisa Bozorgzad, and Azam Saii. 2014. "Effect of Applying Continuous Care Model on Quality of Life among Kidney Transplant Patients: A Randomized Clinical Trial." *Iranian Journal of Kidney Diseases* 8 (2): 139–44.

Rodrigue, James R., Robert Guenther, Bruce Kaplan, Didier A. Mandelbrot, Martha Pavlakis, and Richard J. Howard. 2008. "Measuring the Expectations of Kidney Donors: Initial Psychometric Properties of the Living Donation Expectancies Questionnaire." *Transplantation* 85 (9): 1230–34.

Rogal, Shari S., Douglas Landsittel, Owen Surman, Raymond T. Chung, and Anna Rutherford. 2011. "Pretransplant Depression, Antidepressant Use, and Outcomes of Orthotopic Liver Transplantation: Depression and Liver Transplant Outcomes." *Liver Transplantation: Official Publication of the American Association for the Study of Liver Diseases and the International Liver Transplantation Society* 17 (3): 251–60.

Sawinski, Deirdre, and Jayme E. Locke. 2019. "Kidney Transplantation in A HIV-Positive Recipient." *Clinical Journal of the American Society of Nephrology, CJN* 2215 (Cjn): 14051118.

Schover, Leslie R., Stevan B. Streem, Navdeep Boparai, Kathleen Duriak, and Andrew C. Novick. 1997. "The Psychosocial Impact of Donating a Kidney: Long-Term Follow up From a Urology Based Center." *The Journal of Urology* 157 (5): 1596–1601.

Schulz, Karl-Heinz, and Sylvia Kroencke. 2015. "Psychosocial Challenges before and after Organ Transplantation." *Transplant Research and Risk Management*, 45.

Fidel Kinori, Sara G., Antonio A. Tadeo, Esther C. Campanera, Gemme C. Requena, Crisanto D. Quevedo, and Anna L. Garreta et al. 2015. "Unified Protocol for Psychiatric and Psychological Assessment of Candidates for Transplantation of Organs and Tissues, PSI-CAT." *Rev Psiquiatr Salud Ment* 8 (3).

Shenoy, Akhil. 2019. "The Psychosocial Evaluation of Live Donors." In *Psychosocial Care of End-Stage Organ Disease and Transplant Patients,* 49–59. Cham: Springer International Publishing.

Surman, Owen S. Psychiatric aspects of organ transplantation. Psychiatric Aspects of Organ Transplantation [Published Erratum Appears in *Am J Psychiatry* 1989 Nov;146(11):1523]." 1989. *The American Journal of Psychiatry* 146 (8): 972–82.

Telles-Correia, Diogo, António Barbosa, Inês Mega. 2010. "Personality and transplantation." *Acta Med Port*.23 (4): 655–62.

Thomas, Caroline Venzon, Elisa Kern de Castro, and Ivan Carlos Ferreira Antonello. 2016. "Personality Traits and Clinical/Biochemical Course in the First Year after Kidney Transplant." *Renal Failure* 38 (9): 1383–90.

Twillman, Robert K., Corinne Manetto, David K. Wellisch, and Deane L. Wolcott. 1993. "The Transplant Evaluation Rating Scale. A Revision of the Psychosocial Levels System for Evaluating Organ Transplant Candidates." *Psychosomatics.*

United Network of Organ Sharing and Scientific Registry of Transplant Recipients. Available From: www.unos.org, Accessed April 12, 2019.

Weng, Li-Chueh, Hsiu-Li Huang, Yi-Wen Wang, Wei-Chen Lee, Kang-Hua Chen, and Tsui-Yun Yang. 2014. "The Effect of Self-Efficacy, Depression and Symptom Distress on Employment Status and Leisure Activities of Liver Transplant Recipients." *Journal of Advanced Nursing* 70 (7): 1573–83.

Wirken, Lieke, Henriët van Middendorp, Christina W. Hooghof, Jan Stephan Sanders, Ruth E. Dam, Karlijn A. M. I. van der Pant, Elsbeth C. M. Berendsen, et al. 2017. "Pre-Donation Cognitions of Potential Living Organ Donors: The Development of the Donation Cognition Instrument in Potential Kidney Donors." *Nephrology, Dialysis,*

Transplantation: Official Publication of the European Dialysis and Transplant Association - European Renal Association 32 (3): 573–80.

Zalai, Dora, Lilla Szeifert, and Marta Novak. 2012. "Psychological Distress And Depression İn Patients With Chronic Kidney Disease." *Semin Dial* 25 (428): 1525–139.

Zhang, Sai-Jun, Li-Hua Huang, Yan-Ling Wen, Zhen-Hua Hu, Jing Jin, Li-Hua Shen, and Li-Xia Cai. 2005. "Impact of Personality and Coping Mechanisms on Health Related Quality of Life in Liver Transplantation Recipients." *Hepatobiliary & Pancreatic Diseases International: HBPD INT* 4 (3): 356–59.

Zhu, Yichen, Yifan Zhou, Lei Zhang, Jian Zhang, and Jun Lin. 2017. "Efficacy of Interventions for Adherence to the Immunosuppressive Therapy in Kidney Transplant Recipients: A Meta-Analysis and Systematic Review." *Journal of Investigative Medicine: The Official Publication of the American Federation for Clinical Research* 65 (7): 1049–56.

Zoellner, Tanja, and Andreas Maercker. 2006. "Posttraumatic Growth in Clinical Psychology — A Critical Review and Introduction of a Two Component Model." *Clinical Psychology Review* 26 (5): 626–53.

In: Kidney Transplantation
Editor: Robert C. Morgan

ISBN: 978-1-53619-721-1
© 2021 Nova Science Publishers, Inc.

Chapter 3

DONOR NEPHRECTOMY TECHNIQUES

Ahmet Emin Dogan[1], Sanem Guler Cimen[2], Tarik Kucuk[1] and Sertac Cimen[1]

[1]University of Health Sciences, Diskapi Training and Research Hospital, Department of Urology, Ankara, Turkey
[2]University of Health Sciences, Diskapi Training and Research Hospital, Department of General Surgery, Ankara, Turkey

ABSTRACT

Renal transplantation from a living donor has better results than cadaveric renal transplantation in terms of patient and graft survival rate, quality of life, and cost. Renal transplantation from living donors is performed safely with positive results due to insufficient cadaveric renal supply. The most classic and commonly used donor nephrectomy technique is the open technique performed with a flank lumbotomy incision. Today, this technique has been rapidly replaced by minimally invasive laparoscopic or robot-assisted donor nephrectomy techniques.

This study aims to define the surgical techniques used in living donor nephrectomy, discuss the use and reliability of these techniques in different patient groups, and examine the long-term follow-up results of donors and recipients. There was no significant difference in complication rates, cost-effectiveness, and graft function in patients undergoing laparoscopic donor nephrectomy compared to open donor nephrectomy. On the other hand, renal transplantation centers should offer donors a few different techniques according to their needs and unique circumstances. Laparoscopic donor nephrectomy has become the gold standard technique for suitable living kidney donors in the last decade. However, it should be kept in mind that open, retroperitoneoscopic, robotic, and hand-assisted techniques can be safely applied for donor nephrectomy in the presence of donor-specific risk or limiting factors such as a history of previous abdominal surgery, multiple kidney arteries or veins, or obesity.

Keywords: renal transplantation, laparoscopy, minimally invasive surgical procedures, donor nephrectomy

INTRODUCTION

Renal transplantation from a living donor has better results than cadaveric renal transplantation in terms of patient and graft survival rate, quality of life, and cost [1-3]. The disadvantage of renal transplantation from a living donor is that a healthy individual needs to undergo surgery for their sick relative. Various surgical techniques can be applied to remove the kidney from the living donor. The most classic and commonly used donor nephrectomy technique is the open technique performed with a flank lumbotomy incision. Today, minimally invasive techniques have rapidly started to replace this technique. The most popular of these techniques is transperitoneal laparoscopic donor nephrectomy, first described by Ratner et al. in 1995 [4]. This technique has brought about positive effects such as less pain after surgery, better cosmetic result, and faster return to daily life. It has become a preferred technique by living donors and organ transplantation surgeons for these reasons. It has been suggested that its application in many organ transplantation centers contributes to the increase in renal transplantation from the living donor. Many series published over the years have shown that laparoscopic donor nephrectomy is as safe and effective as open donor nephrectomy [5, 6]. Some changes have occurred in these two techniques in recent years (Table

1). A 2005 study on living donor nephrectomies found that 40% of nephrectomies performed in western Europe were performed laparoscopically, and this rate was 67% in the United States in 2003 [7, 8]. Different surgical techniques associated with laparoscopic donor nephrectomy are discussed in this review.

Table 1. Live Donor Nephrectomy Techniques

Open donor nephrectomy technique
• Classical lumbotomy
• Muscle-sparing mini incision donor nephrectomy
Laparoscopic transperitoneal technique
• Laparoscopic donor nephrectomy
• Hand-assisted laparoscopic donor nephrectomy
Laparoscopic retroperitoneal technique
• Endoscopic retroperitoneal laparoscopic donor nephrectomy
• Endoscopic retroperitoneal hand-assisted laparoscopic donor nephrectomy
Robot Assisted Donor Nephrectomy

SURGERY TECHNIQUES

Open Donor Nephrectomy

Open donor nephrectomy by lumbotomy technique is a classic technique used to obtain renal grafts from living donors for decades. This technique is safe for both donor and renal graft and constitutes the gold standard compared to all new techniques.

The donor is placed in the lateral decubitus position, and the flank area is completely exposed, bringing the operating table from the belly level to flexion. Open donor nephrectomy is performed retroperitoneally with a 15-25 cm flank incision under the 12th rib. Resection of the distal portion of the 12th rib is often necessary to ensure adequate access to the kidney. Gerota's fascia is revealed after the triple abdominal wall muscle layer is incised. The kidney is then released from the surrounding tissues. Renal artery and vein are isolated, ureter with sufficient periureteral tissue is dissected as far as possible and connected. The kidney is quickly removed from the surgical site, and cold perfusion is initiated at the other table after ligating the renal artery and vein. The duration of hot ischemia is relatively short, and the risk of postoperative complications such as adhesion, intestinal perforation, and ileus is low in this technique. However, open donor nephrectomy significantly damages the abdominal wall and causes postoperative pain, long-term hospitalization, and cosmetic problems [9]. Side effects such as denervation of the abdominal wall and incisional hernia may be observed in the long term. These techniques have replaced open donor nephrectomy due to the increasing popularity of minimally invasive techniques in the last decade.

Minimal Invasive Open Donor Nephrectomy

Muscle protective mini-incision open donor nephrectomy has gained popularity for a short period during the transition to laparoscopic nephrectomy, but it is not used today except for particular indications. This operation can be performed with anterior, flank, and posterior approaches with an incision of approximately 7 cm. It is opened with a horizontal skin incision at the 11th rib level after the donor is placed in the lateral decubitus position and the operating table is brought to flexion. The internal oblique and transverse abdominal muscles in the abdominal wall are atraumatically separated without damaging the intercostal nerves. Gerota's fascia is reached after medializing the peritoneal layer with blunt dissection. Long-handled surgical instruments are preferred because of the limited operation area. The kidney is meticulously separated from the surrounding adipose tissues, and subsequently, the arterial and venous structures are isolated. The ureter is dissected until its distal end, ligated, and divided. The kidney is removed immediately after the renal artery and the renal vein is divided. This approach aims to combine the traditional open technique's safety with the advantages of the laparoscopic technique. It has advantages such as less blood loss and shorter hospital stay compared to classic open donor nephrectomy. Also, complications caused by surgical incisions are less common. Only a slight increase in surgical time may be observed [10-12]. Lewis et al. found that blood loss was higher in the open donor nephrectomy technique than the other techniques in their prospective study that compared traditional open, minimally invasive open, and laparoscopic donor nephrectomy methods. Similarly, the need for postoperative intravenous analgesia was found to be higher in open nephrectomy. Besides, minimally invasive open donor nephrectomy led to a slower recovery and lower quality of life score than laparoscopic donor nephrectomy. No significant difference was found between the two techniques regarding graft and donor survival [13-15].

Laparoscopic Transperitoneal Donor Nephrectomy

The table is brought to maximum flexion and entered with 4 or 5 trocars when the donor is in the lateral decubitus position in the laparoscopic transperitoneal donor nephrectomy technique. The abdomen is inflated up to 12 mmHg. The colon is medialized. The Gerota's fascia is opened, and the renovascular pedicle is isolated. Then the adrenal, gonadal, and lumbar veins are clipped and separated. The ureter is clipped and divided from its distal. Pfannenstiel (transverse suprapubic) incision is performed to remove the kidney. The renal artery and vein are divided by endoscopic staplers; the kidney is taken out of the body, perfused with preservation solution, and stored in the cold. Removal of the kidney can be performed directly by hand or with an endoscopic bag. The most crucial disadvantage of this technique is that it requires a long learning period. Also, bowel injuries, development of trocar hernia, and bowel adhesions that may occur during trocar placement are encountered at a similar frequency as in all laparoscopic cases [16]. Cases of a lumbar vein, renal artery, aorta, spleen injury, pneumomediastinum, and hematoma have also been reported [17]. The rate of transition to open surgery has been reported as 1.8%. The transition to open surgery is usually due to bleeding or vascular injury [18].

It seems to be a disadvantage to obtain a short vascular pedicle in the transperitoneal laparoscopic technique when the transperitoneal laparoscopic and open techniques are compared. Besides, hot ischemia and operation time in laparoscopic donor nephrectomy may be slightly longer than open donor nephrectomy. These differences disappear as the experience of the center and surgeon increases in laparoscopic technique. Simforoosh et al. compared the results of open and transperitoneal laparoscopic donor nephrectomy. No difference was found between the techniques in terms of graft survival and complication rates in this study. However, the laparoscopic technique was superior in terms of postoperative satisfaction rates and turning back to normal daily life activities [2]. There are also meta-analyses comparing the two techniques in addition to these studies. These meta-analyses confirm that transperitoneal laparoscopic donor nephrectomy shortens hospital stay duration, reduces the need for postoperative analgesia, and creates better cosmetic results than open donor nephrectomy [15-19]. In some centers routine placement of drains after laparoscopic donor nephrectomy has been suggested but in some studies there was no significant difference between the drain and no drain groups in terms of length of hospital stay, complication rate [20].

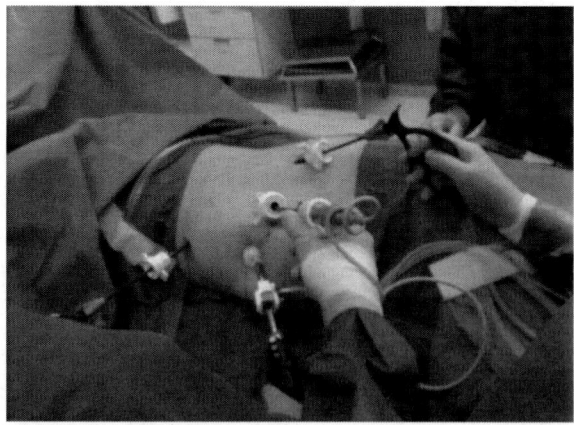

Figure 1. Port placement at the pure laparoscopic donor nephrectomy technique.

Retroperitoneoscopic Donor Nephrectomy

The retroperitoneal endoscopic donor nephrectomy technique was developed to reduce possible intra-abdominal complications in transperitoneal laparoscopic techniques. It is retracted to the medial without opening the peritoneum in this technique. It can be performed technically-assisted or fully retroperitoneoscopically. The retroperitoneal cavity is created with the help of a hand or balloon after the donor is placed in the lateral position and inflated with carbon dioxide so that the pressure is 12 mmHg. The dissection of Gerota's fascia, perirenal tissue, and vascular structures is performed similarly to other techniques. It is a recommended technique, especially in donors with a history of previous abdominal surgery, since it does not require entering the adhesive abdomen.

Hand-Assisted Laparoscopic/Retroperitoneoscopic Donor Nephrectomy

Hand-assisted laparoscopic donor nephrectomy can be performed transperitoneally or retroperitoneally [21]. It is argued that the attached hand port provides additional security compared to full techniques. It is suggested that bleeding can be stopped faster due to the presence of the surgeon's hand in the surgical site. Different incisions such as Pfannenstiel, midline supraumbilical, or periumbilical incision have been described for hand entry. The surgeon inserts the non-dominant hand into the surgical site and creates additional space for two trocars with blunt dissection after the hand port's insertion. The right or left colon is released after abdominal insufflation, the renal pedicle is isolated, and the kidney is released from the surrounding tissues. The surgeon positions the kidney laterally to create traction and medialize the colon or peritoneum during these maneuvers. After the ureter is transected at its distal end, initially the renal artery, and subsequently, the vein is divided, and the kidney is removed from the hand port. The most significant disadvantage for surgeons performing this surgery is the cumbersome position; the surgeon usually has to work in an unfavorable position with a bent waist in this technique. Additionally, numbness and temporary numbness may occur in the surgeon's hand stuck for a long time in the small hand port. The frequent entry of the surgeon's hand through the hand port increases the risk of traumatic tissue damage in this area and causes higher wound infection and incisional hernia formation compared to other techniques.

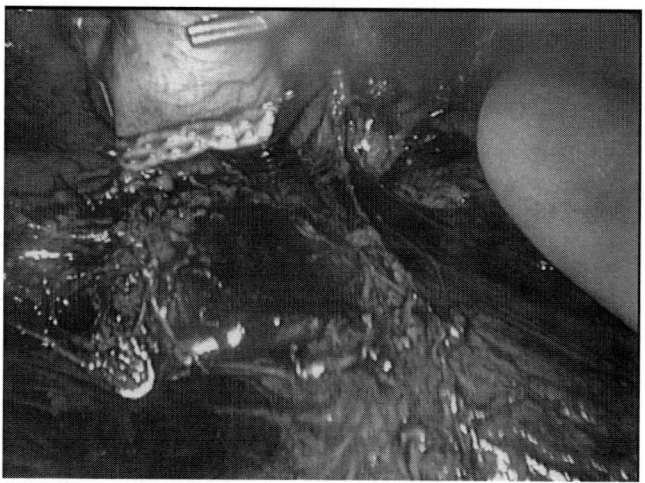

Figure 2. Surgeon's finger, assisting the stapling procedure in a hand assisted laparoscopic donor nephrectomy.

The transition rate to open surgery was reported to be 2.97% in laparoscopic/retroperitoneoscopic donor nephrectomies performed with hand-assisted technique [22]. The most important reasons for the transition to open surgery are intraoperative bleeding, vascular injury, adhesions, and loss of pneumoperitoneum, similar to other techniques. Potential advantages of hand-assisted laparoscopic donor nephrectomy compared to full laparoscopic nephrectomy include less kidney traction, rapid control of bleeding, faster removal of the kidney, and shorter duration of hot ischemia [22, 23]. Kokkinos et al. found that the duration of hot ischemia was shorter in the hand-assisted technique in their meta-analysis comparing full laparoscopic donor nephrectomy and hand-assisted laparoscopic donor nephrectomy. A possible reason for this is that the surgeon, whose hand is already in the operation site, can quickly remove the kidney as soon as the vascular stapling and division is completed. Wolf et al. retrospectively compared the hand-assisted laparoscopy group with the two groups undergoing open donor nephrectomy and found 47% less analgesic need, 35% shorter hospital stay, and 23% earlier return to work-life in the hand-assisted laparoscopy group [24, 25]. Bergmann et al. observed no difference between the hand-assisted laparoscopy group and the full laparoscopy group in a controlled randomized clinical study on intraoperative and postoperative complications [23].

Robot-Assisted Donor Nephrectomy

Robot-assisted donor nephrectomy can be performed as full or hand-assisted. The Da Vinci surgical system consists of 3 components: a console, a control tower, and a surgical arm carrier. Donor nephrectomy is performed while the patient is in the decubitus position, unlike other techniques. The operating table is adjusted so that the kidney can be exposed. Four trocars are placed on the abdomen's left or right side to allow the placement of the three-jointed robotic arm, the robotic camera,

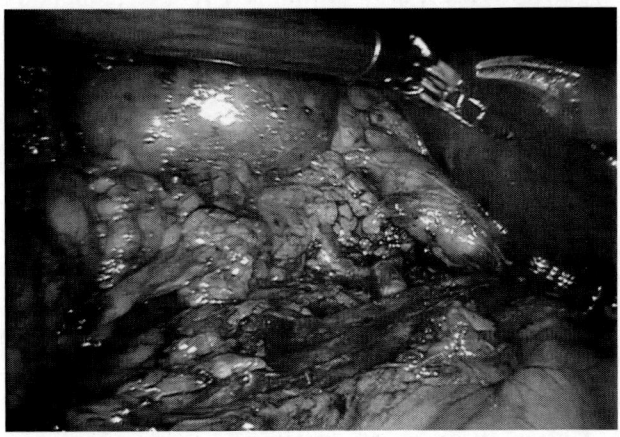

Figure 3. Robot-Assisted Donor Nephrectomy Operation View.

and standard laparoscopic instruments for retraction and dissection during the procedure. The left or right colon is medialized, and the kidney is exposed. Gerota's fascia, perirenal tissue, and vascular structures are dissected. No significant difference was found between the intraoperative and postoperative results between the two techniques in a study conducted with a small number of patients comparing robot-assisted donor nephrectomy and open donor nephrectomy [26]. There is a need for prospective studies on this subject. The advantage of the robot-assisted technique is the freedom of movement brought by the articulation of robot arms. The most significant disadvantage is its high cost.

OPERATIONAL VARIABLES

Donor Nephrectomy Side

A multidisciplinary team in organ transplantation councils should decide which kidney to remove from the living donor. The test results revealing the anatomical, vascular, and even functional structure of the kidneys should be available before this decision. It should not be forgotten in any case that the kidney with better function should be left in the donor. Most centers prefer to use the left kidney. This preference is based on the fact that the left renal vein is approximately 1.5-2 cm longer than the right [27-29]. This extra length helps the surgeon during venous anastomosis, especially in recipients with obese and deep pelvic anatomy. However, some surgeons prefer the right kidney because right colon mobilization can be performed faster, and there is no risk of spleen laceration [30]. A single-center controlled randomized study compared left- and right-sided laparoscopic donor nephrectomies and could not detect a difference in donor quality of life, donor and recipient complication rates, and graft survival. The only significant difference in this study was the duration of surgery, and the duration of the right donor nephrectomy was significantly shorter [31]. The absence of lumbar, adrenal, and gonadal veins participating in the left renal vein is one of the reasons facilitating right renal hilar dissection, in addition to being able to mobilize the right colon more quickly.

Multiple Renal Arteries and Veins

The probability of multiple renal arteries in the kidneys has been reported to be 12-33% [32, 33]. Implantation of kidneys with multiple renal arteries has been associated with vascular and urological complications such as thrombosis and ureteral ischemia. The presence of multiple renal arteries is considered as a relative contraindication by some centers [33, 34]. However, more recent studies have found that the implantation of kidneys with multiple renal arteries can also be performed safely [35-37]. The lower polar accessory artery, which is vital for the lower pole and ureter's blood supply, needs to be preserved. Complications that may require additional surgery, such as ureteral stricture, may occur in the event of thrombosis of this artery. Multiple renal veins are observed in 5-10% of donors [32, 33]. Small accessory renal veins can be securely ligated. However, an accessory vein may be necessary to extend a short right renal vein or to reconstruct a damaged vein. No matter which donor nephrectomy technique is used, multiple renal arteries or veins should not be considered an absolute contraindication for the donor nephrectomy procedure.

Warm Ischemia Time and Duration of Surgery

Warm ischemia time is when the kidney remains at body temperature after its blood supply was blocked. This period is essential because, as a result of the kidney cells' continuing cellular functions, free oxygen radicals accumulate. Accumulated oxygen radicals may cause inflammation of the kidney after reperfusion, causing delayed graft function or primary graft dysfunction. Open nephrectomy comes to the forefront with shorter warm ischemia time than laparoscopic donor nephrectomy [18]. Similarly, shorter warm ischemia times can be recorded in hand-assisted techniques compared to the full laparoscopic donor nephrectomy technique [22]. It was observed that it generally had longer ischemia time than open techniques when Ratner et al. first described the full laparoscopic donor nephrectomy technique; however, warm ischemia times were shortened with increased surgical experience, improvements in laparoscopic surgical instruments as well as concurrent binding and cutting systems in vascular stapler models. Today, the duration of hot ischemia in laparoscopic techniques is almost the same as in open technique. On the other hand, it was found that the total duration of hot ischemia, which was less than 10 minutes, had no adverse effect on graft function [38]. In almost all laparoscopic series, this time is less than 10 minutes.

Elderly Donors

It is basic physiological information that the number of nephrons in the kidney gradually decreases with aging. A healthy 90-year-old person has approximately 30-50% less kidney volume and glomerular number than a 30-year-old person. However, elderly living kidneys, which are also defined marginally, can be used to reduce the mortality rates in the kidney transplantation waiting list. While donors older than 45 were previously defined as elderly donors, currently, donors older than 60 are considered elderly donors [39].

Preoperative evaluation gains more importance in living elderly donors as comorbidities such as hypertension and diabetes increase with advanced age. Renal transplantation from elderly donors was associated with early renal hyperfiltration, delayed graft function, and short-term graft survival in clinical studies [40, 41]. However, this patient group is more advantageous in terms of survival and quality of life than patients who have to continue dialysis.

Garg et al. reported that advanced age during weight was associated with decreased glomerular filtration rate (GFR) before and after donation [42]. Boudville et al. found an increase of 5 mmHg in post-transplant blood pressure compared to the increase predicted with normal aging [43]. Donor age does not constitute a contraindication for living transplantations. It is necessary to evaluate each donor individually. Also, the recipient should be informed about the long-term results related to marginal graft [44].

Obese Donors

Obesity is a global health problem. 15% of women were classified as obese and 40% as overweight in 2016, according to the World Health Organization (WHO) data. In males, this rate was 11% and 39%, respectively. Transplant centers are increasingly facing obese donors in line with these statistics. Also, obesity is considered an independent cardiovascular risk factor and a significant risk factor for all postoperative complications, including living renal transplantation [45, 46]. Obesity is now considered an independent risk factor for end-stage renal failure alone [47]. Obese people are at higher risk of end-stage renal failure compared to normal-weight individuals. Praga et al. observed in a retrospective study of 73 diseases that 13 (92%) of 14 obese donors and 12% of non-obese donors developed proteinuria and renal failure at the end of 10 years of follow-up [48]. It was shown in a retrospective study involving a total of 5304 donors that there was no difference between normal weight and obese donors in terms of re-hospitalization and re-operation rates.

Obese donors can be considered viable donors if no contraindication is observed after detailed clinical evaluation despite the adverse effects of obesity described above. This detailed clinical evaluation should cover the cardiovascular system, respiratory system, and endocrine system and carefully reveal individualized risk factors. Besides, donors should be advised to lose weight and encouraged to adopt a healthy lifestyle before donation [44].

There are studies suggesting that minimally invasive techniques reduce the morbidity of obese donors in terms of donor nephrectomy techniques. Small surgical incisions in minimally invasive techniques significantly reduce the risk of postoperative surgical site infection. Also, the decrease in the need for postoperative analgesia reduced the incidence of the rarely encountered ileus. Some centers applying the minimally invasive technique have reported that they modify the surgical techniques according to the donor's body mass index. These modifications may occur in patient position, trocar placement, targeted intra-abdominal pressure, and dissection plan areas. Renal removal is recommended with different surgical techniques adapted to the living donor instead of a single surgical technique suitable for each living donor.

POST-OPERATIVE VARIABLES

Complications

The defined mortality risk for open and laparoscopic donor nephrectomy is 0.03% [8, 49]. The complication rate of donor nephrectomy has been reported to be 10% [6, 18]. Complications of Clavien-Dindo grade 3 and above are rare, and their frequency varies between 2.9-5.8% [51-53]. Those caused by pulmonary and immobilization among these complications are significantly reduced when a minimally invasive technique is used. Especially atelectasis, pneumothorax, pulmonary congestion, hypoxia, thrombophlebitis, intramural thrombus, and deep vein thrombosis have been reported much less in laparoscopic donor nephrectomy compared to open technique.

Long-Term Follow-Up

Today, long-term kidney donor follow-ups have revealed that giving kidneys to healthy people who are suitable to be kidney donors does not shorten life and does not cause deterioration in life quality [54, 55]. Similarly, it was observed in the 45-year follow-up of World War II veterans that the risk of hypertension and end-stage renal failure did not increase [56]. Kidney disease was reported to develop in 11 donors during the long-term follow-up of 3698 kidney donors in a single-center clinical study [57]. This rate is 268/1000000 people in the general population. Also, living kidney donors were found to have a higher quality of life than the control group. Living kidney donors should be followed up by organ transplantation centers in the long term regardless of the surgical technique used. They should be periodically screened for early disease markers such as high blood pressure, glucose intolerance, and proteinuria. Preventive measures should be taken immediately in case of detection of these markers. Not harming the organ donor should be the main target of the organ transplantation center [58].

Recipient Kidney Function

After laparoscopic donor nephrectomy and open donor nephrectomy, one-year graft survival rates were reported to be between 93-100% and 91-100%, respectively [6, 18]. Five-year graft survival after laparoscopic donor nephrectomy and open donor nephrectomy has been reported as 91% and 86%, respectively [19]. There are no long-term data comparing laparoscopic donor nephrectomy and open donor nephrectomy technique in terms of long-term graft survival. It can be concluded with the current clinical data that laparoscopic removal of living donor kidneys has no clinically measurable negative effect on renal transplantation. However, these successful results depend on the careful and multidisciplinary evaluation of viable kidney donor candidates so that only healthy and motivated individuals can become living donors.

Cost

It can be thought that the laparoscopic technique may be more expensive because the tools used in laparoscopic donor nephrectomy are more expensive and have a limited number of uses when the surgical costs of laparoscopic and open donor nephrectomy techniques are compared.

However, it is observed that these costs are equalized considering the shortened length of hospital stay when the laparoscopic method is used, decreased complication rate, and early return to work [6, 59]. This cost analysis gradually shifts in favor of the laparoscopic technique, especially in experienced centers.

CONCLUSION

Laparoscopic donor nephrectomy gained popularity, especially among living donors, after it was first defined in 1995 and demanded by organ transplantation centers. It has become widespread among surgeons to increase the living donor pool and has been the most commonly used donor nephrectomy method in recent years, considering the demands. Modifications of the technique were developed, and its reliability increased as the experience increased. The laparoscopic donor nephrectomy technique results were similar to the open nephrectomy technique in terms of graft survival in long-term clinical studies. Again, variations such as the right donor kidney, multiple renal arteries, or veins have not also been a reason for hesitation with increasing experience. Laparoscopic donor nephrectomy has been shown to have superior results regarding postoperative pain, cosmetic condition, recovery, and return to daily activities compared to open donor nephrectomy. There is no significant difference between the two approaches in terms of complication rates, cost-effectiveness, and graft function. Today, laparoscopic donor nephrectomy has become a standard and preferred donor surgery method for renal transplantation from living donors in many centers.

REFERENCES

[1] Fonouni H, Mehrabi A, Golriz M, et al. Comparison of the laparoscopic versus open live donor nephrectomy: an overview of

surgical complications and outcome. *Langenbecks Arch Surg* (2014) 399:543–551.

[2] Simforoosh N, Basiri A, Tabibi A, et al. Comparison of laparoscopic and open donor nephrectomy: a randomized controlled trial. *BJU Int.* 2005;95(6):851-5.

[3] Cadeddu JA, Ratner L, Kavoussi LR. Laparoscopic donor nephrectomy. *Semin Laparosc Surg.* 2000 Sep;7(3):195-9.

[4] Ratner LE, Ciseck LJ, Moore RG, Cigarroa FG, Kaufman HS, Kavoussi LR. Laparoscopic live donor nephrectomy. *Transplantation.* 1995;60(9):1047-9.

[5] Shokeir AA. Open versus laparoscopic live donor nephrectomy: a focus on the safety of donors and the need for a donor registry. *J Urol.* 2007;178(5):1860-6.

[6] Tooher RL, Rao MM, Scott DF, et al. A systematic review of laparoscopic live-donor nephrectomy. *Transplantation.* 2004; 78(3):404-14.

[7] Kok NF, Weimar W, Alwayn IP, IJzermans JN. The current practice of live donor nephrectomy in Europe. *Transplantation.* 2006;82(7):892-7.

[8] Matas AJ, Bartlett ST, Leichtman AB, Delmonico FL. Morbidity and mortality after living kidney donation, 1999-2001: survey of United States transplant centers. *Am J Transplant.* 2003;3(7):830-4.

[9] Srivastava A, Tripathi DM, Zaman W, Kumar A. Subcostal versus transcostal mini donor nephrectomy: is rib resection responsible for pain related donor morbidity. *J Urol.* 2003;170(3):738-40.

[10] Kok NF, Alwayn IP, Schouten O, Tran KT, Weimar W, IJzermans JN. Mini-incision open donor nephrectomy as an alternative to classic lumbotomy: evolution of the open approach. *Transpl Int.* 2006;19(6):500-5.

[11] Lewis GR, Brook NR, Waller JR, Bains JC, Veitch PS, Nicholson ML. A comparison of traditional open, minimal-incision donor nephrectomy and laparoscopic donor nephrectomy. *Transpl Int.* 2004;17(10):589-95.

[12] Schnitzbauer AA, Kaybı M, Hornung M, Glockzin G, Mantouvalou L, Krüger B, Krämer BK, Schlitt HJ, A Obed Mini-incision for strictly retroperitoneal nephrectomy in living kidney donation vs flank incision. *Nephrol Dial Transplant.* 2006 Oct;21(10):2948-52.

[13] Kok NF, Lind MY, Hansson BM, et al. Comparison of laparoscopic and mini incision open donor nephrectomy: single blind, randomised controlled clinical trial. *BMJ.* 2006;333(7561):221.

[14] Kok NF, Alwayn IP, Tran KT, Hop WC, Weimar W, IJzermans JN. Psychosocial and physical impairment after mini-incision open and laparoscopic donor nephrectomy: A prospective study. *Transplantation.* 2006;82(10):1291-7.

[15] Kanashiro Hideki, Lopes Roberto Iglesias, Saito Fernando Akira, Gönye Anuar İbrahim, Denes Francisco Tibor, Chambô José Luis, Falci Renato Jr, Piovesan Affonso Celso, Neto Elias David, Nahas William Carlos. Comparison between laparoscopic and subcostal mini-incision for live donor nephrectomy. *Einstein (Sao Paulo).* 2010 Dec;8(4):456-60.

[16] 16-)Oyen O, Andersen M, Mathisen L, et al. Laparoscopic versus open living-donor nephrectomy: experiences from a prospective, randomized, single-center study focusing on donor safety. *Transplantation.* 2005;79(9):1236-40

[17] Leventhal JR, Kocak B, Salvalaggio PR, et al. Laparoscopic donor nephrectomy 1997 to 2003: lessons learned with 500 cases at a single institution. *Surgery.* 2004;136(4):881-90.

[18] Nanidis TG, Antcliffe D, Kokkinos C, et al. Laparoscopic versus open live donor nephrectomy in renal transplantation: a meta-analysis. *Ann Surg.* 2008;247(1):58-70.

[19] Uysal Erdal, Yüzbaşioğlu M. Fatih, Dokur Mehmet, Sipahi Mesut, Aksoy Başar. Comparison of Laparoscopic and Open Donor Nephrectomy on Living Donor Renal Transplantations. *Bozok Tıp Derg.* 2015;5(4):1-6.

[20] Celasin H, Kocaay AF, Cimen SG. *Surgical Drains After Laparoscopic Donor Nephrectomy: Needed or Not?*

[21] Maartense S, Idu M, Bemelman FJ, Balm R, Surachno S, Bemelman WA. Hand-assisted laparoscopic live donor nephrectomy. *Br J Surg.* 2004;91(3):344-8.

[22] Kokkinos C, Nanidis T, Antcliffe D, Darzi AW, Tekkis P, Papalois V. Comparison of laparoscopic versus hand-assisted live donor nephrectomy. *Transplantation.* 2007;83(1):41-7.

[23] Bargman V, Sundaram CP, Bernie J, Goggins W. Randomized trial of laparoscopic donor nephrectomy with and without hand assistance. *J Endourol.* 2006;20(10):717-22.

[24] El-Galley R, Hood N, Young CJ, Deierhoi M, Urban DA. Donor nephrectomy: A comparison of techniques and results of open, hand assisted and full laparoscopic nephrectomy. *J Urol.* 2004;171(1):40-3.

[25] Wolf JS, Jr., Merion RM, Leichtman AB, et al. Randomized controlled trial of hand-assisted laparoscopic versus open surgical live donor nephrectomy. *Transplantation.* 2001;72(2):284-90.

[26] Leonienke F. C. Dols Niels F. M. Kok Jan N. M. IJzermans. Live donor nephrectomy: a review of evidence for surgical techniques. *Transpl Int.* 2010 Feb;23(2):121-30.

[27] Lennerling A, Blohme I, Ostraat O, Lonroth H, Olausson M, Nyberg G. Laparoscopic or open surgery for living donor nephrectomy. N*ephrol Dial Transplant.* 2001;16(2):383-6.

[28] Toshiaki Kashiwadate, Kazuaki Tokodai, Noritoshi Amada, Izumi Haga, Tetsuro Takayama, Atsushi Nakamura, Takuya Jimbo, Yasuyuki Hara, Naoki Kawagishi, Noriaki Ohuchi. Right versus left retroperitoneoscopic living-donor nephrectomy. *Int Urol Nephrol.* 2015 Jul;47(7):1117-21.

[29] Kumar A, Chaturvedi S, Gulia A, Maheshwari R, Dassi V, Desai P. Laparoscopic Live Donor Nephrectomy: Comparison of Outcomes Right Versus Left. *Transplant Proc.* 2018 Oct;50(8):2327-2332.

[30] Lind MY, Hazebroek EJ, Hop WC, Weimar W, Jaap BH, Ijzermans JN. Right-sided laparoscopic live donor nephrectomy: is reluctance stil justified? *Transplantation.* 2002;74(7):1045-8.

[31] Minnee RC, Bemelman WA, Maartense S, Bemelman FJ, Gouma DJ, Idu MM. Left or right kidney in hand-assisted donor nephrectomy? A randomized controlled trial. *Transplantation.* 2008;85(2):203-8.

[32] Grant I S Disick, Michael E Shapiro, Ruth Ann Miles, Ravi Munver. Critical analysis of laparoscopic donor nephrectomy in the setting of complex renal vasculature: initial experience and intermediate outcomes. *J Endourol.* 2009 Mar;23(3):451-5.

[33] Roza AM, Perloff LJ, Naji A, Grossman RA, Barker CF. Living-related donors with bilateral multiple renal arteries. A twenty-year experience. *Transplantation.* 1989;47(2):397-9.

[34] Guerra EE, Didone EC, Zanotelli ML, et al. Renal transplants with multiple arteries. *Transplant Proc.* 1992;24(5):1868.

[35] Kok NF, Dols LF, Hunink MG, et al. Complex vascular anatomy in live kidney donation: imaging and consequences for clinical outcome. *Transplantation.* 2008;85(12):1760-5.

[36] li-El-Dein B, Osman Y, Shokeir AA, Shehab El-Dein AB, Sheashaa H, Ghoneim MA. Multiple arteries in live donor renal transplantation: surgical aspects and outcomes. *J Urol.* 2003; 169(6):2013 7.

[37] Minnee RC, Surachno S, Bemelman F, et al. Impact of additional vascular reconstructions on survival of kidney transplants. *Int Surg.* 2008;93(2):111-5.

[38] Simforoosh N, Basiri A, Shakhssalim N, Ziaee SA, Tabibi A, Moghaddam SM. Effect of warm ischemia on graft outcome in laparoscopic donor nephrectomy. *J Endourol.* 2006;20(11):895-8.

[39] P. Di Cocco, G. Orlando, V. Rizza, L. De Luca, M. D'Angelo, K. Clemente, A. Famulari, and F. Pisani. Kidney Transplantation From Older Donors. *Transplant Proc.* 2011 May;43(4):1033-5.

[40] K Noppakun [1], FG Cosio, PG Dean, et al. Living donor age and kidney transplant outcomes. *Am J Transplant.* 2011 Jun;11(6):1279-86.

[41] Sanchez-Fructuoso AI, Prats D, Marques M, et al. Does renal mass exert an independent effect on the determinants of antigen-dependent injury? *Transplantation.* 2001;71(3):381-6.

[42] Garg AX, Muirhead N, Knoll G, et al. Proteinuria and reduced kidney function in living kidney donors: A systematic review, meta-analysis, and meta-regression. *Kidney Int.* 2006;70(10):1801-10.

[43] Boudville N, Prasad GV, Knoll G, et al. Meta-analysis: risk for hypertension in living kidney donors. *Ann Intern Med* 2006;145(3):185-96.

[44] British Transplantation Society, *The Renal Association. United Kingdom guidelines for living donor kidney transplantation* (second edition). 1-4-2005. Internet.

[45] Heimbach JK, Taler SJ, Prieto M, et al. Obesity in living kidney donors: clinical characteristics and outcomes in the era of laparoscopic donor nephrectomy. *Am J Transplant.* 2005;5(5):1057-64.

[46] Pesavento TE, Henry ML, Falkenhain ME, et al. Obese living kidney donors: short-term results and possible implications. *Transplantation.* 1999;68(10):1491-6.

[47] Hsu CY, McCulloch CE, Iribarren C, et al. Body mass index and risk for end-stage renal disease. *Ann Intern Med.* 2006;144(1):21-8.

[48] Praga M, Hernandez E, Herrero JC, et al. Influence of obesity on the appearance of proteinuria and renal insufficiency after unilateral nephrectomy. *Kidney Int.* 2000;58(5):2111-8.

[49] Najarian JS, Chavers BM, McHugh LE, Matas AJ. 20 years or more of follow-up of living kidney donors. *Lancet.* 1992;340(8823):807-10.

[50] Clavien PA, Camargo CA, Jr., Croxford R, Langer B, Levy GA, Greig PD. Definition and classification of negative outcomes in solid organ transplantation. Application in liver transplantation. *Ann Surg.* 1994;220(2):109-20.

[51] Mjoen G, Oyen O, Holdaas H, Midtvedt K, Line PD. Morbidity and mortality in 1022 consecutive living donor nephrectomies: benefits of a living donor registry. *Transplantation.* 2009;88(11):1273-9.

[52] Patel S, Cassuto J, Orloff M, et al. Minimizing morbidity of organ donation: analysis of factors for perioperative complications after living-donor nephrectomy in the United States. *Transplantation.* 2008;85(4):561-5.

[53] Permpongkosol S, Link RE, Su LM, et al. Complications of 2,775 urological laparoscopic procedures: 1993 to 2005. *J Urol.* 2007; 177(2):580-5.

[54] Benjamin R. Morgan and Hassan N. Ibrahim. Long-term outcomes of kidney donors. *Current Opinion in Nephrology and Hypertension* 2011, 20:605–609.

[55] Fehrman-Ekholm I, Elinder CG, Stenbeck M, Tyden G, Groth CG. Kidney donors live longer. *Transplantation.* 1997;64(7):976-8.

[56] Narkun-Burgess DM, Nolan CR, Norman JE, Page WF, Miller PL, Meyer TW. Forty-five year follow-up after uninephrectomy. *Kidney Int.* 1993;43(5):1110-5.

[57] Ibrahim HN, Foley R, Tan L, et al. Long-term consequences of kidney donation. *N Engl J Med.* 2009;360(5):459-69.

[58] El-Agroudy Amgad E, Sabry Alaa A, Wafa Ehab W, et al. Long-term follow-up of living kidney donors: a longitudinal study. Mohamed A Ghoneim. *BJU Int.* 2007 Aralık; 100 (6): 1351-5.

[59] Kok NF, Adang EM, Hansson BM, et al. Cost effectiveness of laparoscopic versus mini-incision open donor nephrectomy: a randomized study. *Transplantation.* 2007;83(12):1582-7.

In: Kidney Transplantation
Editor: Robert C. Morgan

ISBN: 978-1-53619-721-1
© 2021 Nova Science Publishers, Inc.

Chapter 4

NEPHRECTOMY TIMING FOR POLYCYSTIC KIDNEYS IN AUTOSOMAL DOMINANT POLYCYSTIC KIDNEY DISEASE PATIENTS LISTED FOR TRANSPLANTATION

Görkem Özenç[1], Sanem Guler Cimen[2] and Sertac Cimen[1]
[1]University of Health Sciences, Diskapi Training and Research Hospital, Department of Urology, Ankara, Turkey
[2]University of Health Sciences, Diskapi Training and Research Hospital, Department of General Surgery, Ankara, Turkey

ABSTRACT

Autosomal dominant polycystic kidney disease (ADPCKD) is a common hereditary disorder causing end-stage renal disease in approximately 10% of the population worldwide. Its symptoms occur in the third and fourth decades of life, due to kidney enlargement and deformation, subsequently leading to renal failure. The definitive treatment of ADPCKD does not exist and current treatment regimens focus on managing the symptoms.

For end-stage renal disease, the best treatment, providing a higher quality of life and overall survival is kidney transplantation. Kidney transplant outcomes are even better with live kidney donations. With live kidney donors, the timing of transplant can be planned and variables can be adjusted to achieve optimal conditions. One of these variables is caused by enlarged and deformed kidneys. These enlarged kidneys may trouble the transplant process by intra-cystic bleeding, infections, stone formations, and mechanical compression of other organs. Additionally, when enlarged below the iliac crest, these kidneys may occupy the space needed for the transplanted kidney. Thus, management of the polycystic kidneys at the pre-transplant period is curial. The decision to remove them, whether to remove single or both kidneys, and the timing of this surgery may affect the outcome of the kidney transplantation significantly.

Keywords: polycystic, kidney, transplantion, nephrectomy

AUTOSOMAL DOMINANT POLYCYSTIC KIDNEY DISEASE

Autosomal Dominant Polycystic Kidney Disease (ADPKD) is one of the most common inherited kidney diseases with a prevalence of 1 / 400-1000 (1). It is responsible for 8-10% of end-stage renal failure (ESRD) cases worldwide [1]. Therefore, it leads to significant mortality and morbidity.

In approximately 85% of cases, the responsible gene is in the short arm of chromosome 16 (16p13.3). This gene is called the PKD1 (Polycystic Kidney Disease 1) gene. In the remaining patients, the genetic defect is in the long arm of chromosome 4 (4q13-23), called the PKD2 gene. Mutations of two major genes cause ADPKD by stimulating renal tubule cells to proliferate at increased rates. Molecular mechanism and/or defective development and function of the primary cilia are involved in causing cysts to form in the kidneys and in the liver. In the late stages, cysts virtually replace the renal parenchyma (Figure 1 and Figure 2 Pathology). In patients carrying PKD1, the age of onset of the disease, hypertension, and the time to develop an end-stage renal disease are shorter than those with PKD2 [2].

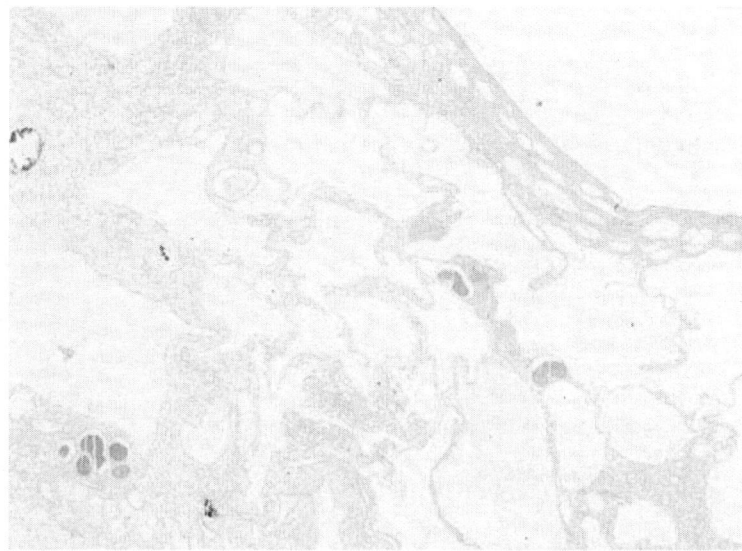

Figure 1. (See Figure 2 caption).

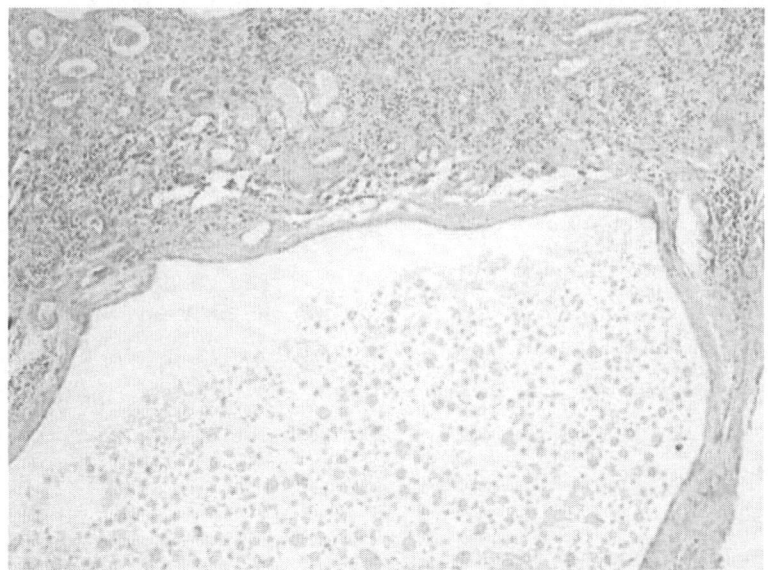

Figure 2. In ADPCKD the renal cysts are lined by cuboidal or flattened epithelium. Areas of global sclerosis, tubular atrophy, interstitial fibrosis and chronic inflammation can also be observed. (H&E stain x4).

In autosomal dominant polycystic kidney disease, both kidneys are large and contain multiple, various-sized cysts (Figure 3). Although the kidneys grow, they often retain their anatomical shape. Sometimes the kidneys can enlarge enough to cover the entire abdomen.

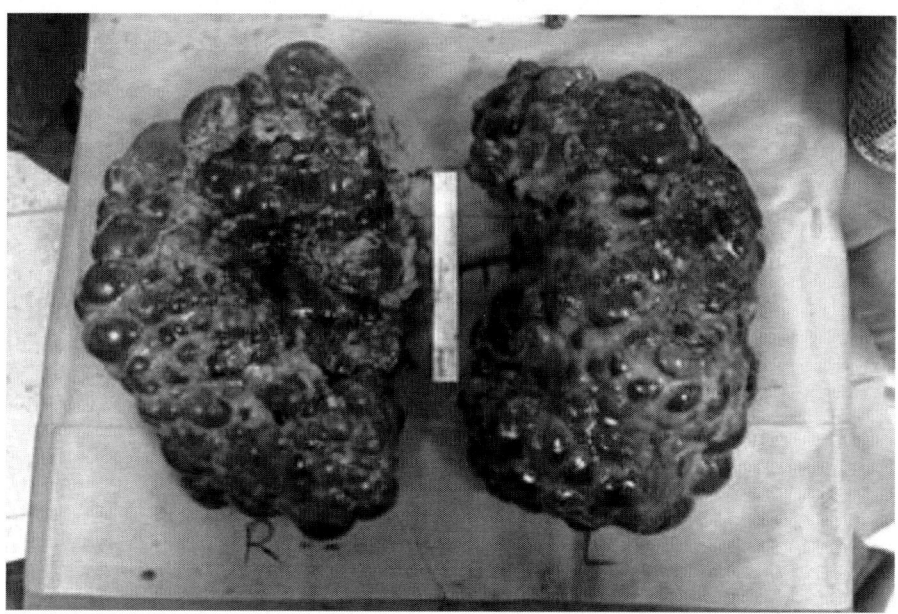

Figure 3. Macroscopic View of Polycystic Kidneys (ADPKD) After Bilateral Native Nephrectomy.

Patients are usually asymptomatic at an early age, although the frequency of symptoms increases with advancing age. In the majority, symptoms occur in the 3rd- 4th decade of life. The most common symptoms are pain, hematuria, urinary tract infections, and uncontrolled hypertension. The most common cause of presentation is flank pain. With the increase in kidney size, compression effect on surrounding organs, bleeding into the cyst, infection, and stone formation may lead to pain. Kidney stones are present in 20–30% of patients with ADPKD [3]. Gastrointestinal symptoms are also recorded due to the mechanical compression of kidneys to adjacent organs.

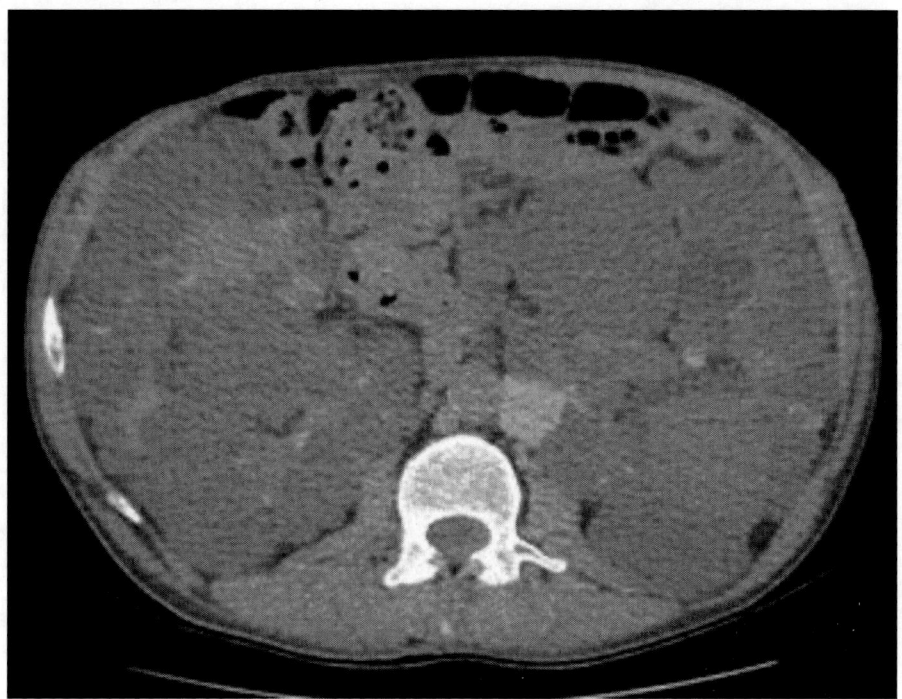

Figure 4. Polycystic Kidneys (ADPKD) CT Abdomen Transvers View.

Renal cell carcinoma (RCC) is not common in ADPKD (< 1% of cases) [4]. However, Hajj et al., compared the prevalence of renal cell carcinoma in patients with chronic renal failure due to ADPKCD and concluded that it was 2-3 times higher in this patient group [5]. Thus, computed tomography follow-up of these cysts is recommended (Figure 4 CT).

Deaths from the ADPKD are mainly due to complications of uremia, arterial hypertension, or intracranial aneurysmal rupture. Treatment that slows or stops the progression is not yet available.

The median age of ESRD development in ADPKDD patients is ten years less than the general ESRD population and was recorded as 54 years [6]. The renal replac ement therapy providing the best survival, rehabilitation, and economical treatment in ESRD patients is kidney transplantation.

PRE-TRANSPLANT EVALUATION

Pre-transplant issues for the ADPKD population differ from patients with other kidney diseases. For example, intracystic bleeding may cause hematuria and contribute to chronic disease anemia. Correcting the anemia may require several blood transfusions. However, as alloimmunization may develop during blood transfusions, transfusions should be avoided unless emergent or life-threatening. Otherwise, anemia should be treated with erythropoietin and iron replacements.

Due to the inherited nature of ADPKD, affected individuals have, on average, only half of the potential living donors than those with non-hereditary kidney disease. Besides, the need for living donors is higher due to the disease burden on the family. Blood group incompatibility also restricts the number of donor candidates. Recipients require counseling to evaluate the live donors carefully within the extended family.

When a family history of ADPKD is determined, potential donors should be screened to guarantee they are free of disease. The age-related ultrasound criteria for both diagnosis and exclusion of the disease are present. However, renal ultrasonography has a sensitivity of only 67% in patients with PKD2 under 30 years of age [7]. The diagnostic sensitivity in patients with PKD1 mutation is approximately 90% between the ages of 15-30, and 100% for older patients. In contrast, diagnostic criteria for other imaging modalities such as MRI or CT with higher resolution for kidney cysts have not been established. Genetic testing can be used in cases when ultrasound is suspicious or proves no cysts and in younger donors (20-40 years old). Expanding live donor exchange programs is another way to increase the options for getting a live donor kidney transplant.

In addition to routine pre-transplant evaluation, ADPKD patients require special consideration: the kidney dimensions with cysts, and potential implications related to recurrent upper urinary tract infections, bleeding, and mechanical compression. For the evaluation of mechanical compression, the physical examination is the first step. Traditionally, if a hand fist can fir in the iliac fossa where the kidney will be placed confirms presence of sufficient space at the iliac fossa. On the other hand, a CT image, showing polycystic kidneys extending below the iliac crest is suggestive of inadequate space for the graft placement.

Another point to consider is the screening of intracranial aneurysms. These aneurysms have been detected in 6% of ADPKD patients who have no family history, and in 20% of patients with a positive family history [8]. Aneurysmal rupture is a feared complication with a mortality rate of 60%. Since magnetic resonance angiography does not require gadolinium, it is used safely for donor evaluations for aneurism screening [9]. According to some studies, cerebral angiographic-MRI scanning provides a more accurate diagnosis in patients younger than 50-55 years with a family history of intracranial aneurysm. Screening is not recommended for asymptomatic patients over 60 [10].

Colonic complications after renal transplantation are rare but have a high mortality rate. Patients with polycystic kidney disease have a significantly higher rate of complicated diverticulitis than other transplant patients. Colon scanning has been recommended in patients over 50 years before transplantation to reduce the impact of colonic diverticular disease. However, Maccune et al., showed that pre-transplant colonoscopic evaluation did not reduce the risk of post-transplant gastrointestinal complications [11]. There is no consensus in the literature for gastrointestinal examination in patients with ADPKDD before transplantation.

Native Nephrectomy of Renal Transplant Recipients with Autosomal-Dominant Polycystic Kidney Disease

Treatment of ADPKD aims at alleviating the symptoms rather than changing the course of the disease or slowing the formation of cysts. However, surgery is often required to overcome (figure intra-op kidneys with cysts) kidney-related complications. The necessity, indication, and especially the timing of nephrectomy in ADPKCD patients scheduled for kidney transplantation are all debatable. This debate can create an intricate problem and a challenge for both the transplant surgeon and the recipient.

Indications for Native Nephrectomy

There is no clear guideline regarding the indications for nephrectomy in patients, but three distinctive categories should be highlighted. First, a native nephrectomy should be considered for patients with chronic pain and gastrointestinal symptoms due to compression of enlarged kidneys, recurrent urinary tract infections, frequent cyst bleeding, and uncontrolled hypertension. If the enlarged multicystic kidneys extending to the pelvis prevent obtaining sufficient space for kidney transplantation, nephrectomy is recommended to recipients scheduled for transplantation. Finally, nephrectomy is advocated for removing a cystic lesion suspicious of malignancy. A literature review shows that timing and indications of native nephrectomy vary widely among transplant centers [12].

NEPHRECTOMY PROCEDURES

The timing and indication for native nephrectomy in patients with ADPKD raise some controversies. In general, surgical procedures have their advantages and disadvantages same applies to native nephrectomy.

In the 1970s, bilateral nephrectomy was preferred prior to kidney transplantation because it reduces complications related to infections [13]. However, the disadvantage of pre-transplant bilateral native nephrectomy is that patients are left anephric and anuric. As a result, patients become dependent on dialysis. If a live donor kidney transplantation is not an option, dialysis can last for months or even years before receiving a transplant on the waitlist. Dialysis diminishes the quality of life and is associated with higher mortality in ESRD patients [14]. Unilateral nephrectomy may be the more appropriate approach for pre-transplant nephrectomy in the absence of a living donor. While the less functional and more problematic kidney is removed, residual diuresis can be preserved, opening space for future kidney transplantation. Although this approach seems beneficial for the recipient, there may be a need for a contralateral native nephrectomy in the future due to mechanical complaints or cyst infections, and this may pose a significant risk for the graft. Whether performed unilaterally or bilaterally, the need for blood transfusions during native nephrectomy prior to transplantation may cause allo-immunization leading to graft rejection. Another disadvantage of pre-transplant nephrectomy is the need for more than one surgical operation.

One of the advantages of native nephrectomy during or after transplantation is the prevention of anephric state and its complications such as anemia, renal osteodystrophy, hyperkalemia, and hypervolemia. Another advantage for the recipients is going through a single operation to get two procedures done.

Nevertheless, simultaneous nephrectomy with transplantation carries risks. These risks include intra-abdominal sepsis secondary to an infected cyst rupture, delay or cancellation of the transplant due to recipient instability, prolonged anesthesia, hypotension due to the removal of giant polycystic kidneys, hypo-perfusion of the allograft, and increased intraoperative blood loss.

One disadvantage of post-transplant native nephrectomy is the delay in postoperative wound healing and increased incisional hernia risk. There is also a risk of infection, which can be more challenging to treat under immunosuppressive therapy. Large polycystic kidneys may compress the transplanted kidney mechanically, resulting in impairment of graft perfusion or ureter strictures [15]. Post-transplant native nephrectomy itself also possesses an austere risk to the graft as intraoperative bleeding and hypotension may lead to graft hypo-perfusion or even arterial thrombosis.

Several issues should be addressed in the decision-making: the importance of residual diuresis, prolonged surgery time, and cold ischemia time. Higher complication rates due to a combined approach, future problems related to the remaining polycystic kidney should be considered.

Literature review shows unilateral or bilateral native nephrectomy before transplantation to be a suitable option for symptomatic ADPKD patients. However, it is imperative to follow suit with a kidney transplant. The patient becomes dialysis-dependent, and longer dialysis duration harms both the patient and graft survival [16, 17].

If live donor kidney transplantation is available, a simultaneous transplant should be scheduled as recommended by Kramer et al. and Fuller et al. Another parameter to be taken into account is **patients'** overall satisfaction and comfort. Glansman et al., evaluated satisfaction in kidney transplant recipients and reported relatively high (70%) satisfaction rates. Although the complication rate was reported to be higher in the simultaneous approach, recipients who underwent renal transplantation alone wished to have this option presented to them [18].

On the other hand, some studies argue that it is wise to avoid any pre-transplant or concurrent procedure. These studies found the estimated percentage of patients with ADPKD requiring native nephrectomy to be relatively low (about 20%) and suggest that patients may not need an extra nephrectomy procedure before or in concomitant kidney transplantation [19, 20].

The selection of the surgical technique is also a controversial issue, the hand-assisted laparoscopic approach is becoming more and more prominently reported in the literature. Although technically challenging, numerous clinical reports, including a recent meta-analysis, have shown that laparoscopic nephrectomy, particularly hand-assisted bilateral nephrectomy, is safe and effective even for very enlarged kidneys [21, 22]. Among the emerging techniques for performing nephrectomy in ADPKD patients, robot-assisted procedures are proven to be efficacious, without major complications, and lower blood loss [23].

Unfortunately, literature consists of retrospectively collected data, and highly variable study designs, making it difficult to reach conclusions. Subsequently, there is no consensus on the appropriate timing for native nephrectomy in patients with ADPKD. Nephrectomy in ADPKD patients who are transplant candidates is a rapidly developing topic, affected by minimally invasive surgery and technological developments in transplantation. The optimal timing and type of surgery are controversial, and more clinical studies and data are needed to determine the best treatment method.

Table 1.

Timing of Native Nephrectomy	Risks	Benefits
Pre-Transplant	<ul><li>Increased need for transfusions (alloimmunization)</li><li>Loss of residual diuresis</li><li>Initiation of dialysis</li><li>Renal osteodystrophy</li><li>Increased risk of hyperkalemia, hypomagnesemia and hypervolemia</li></ul>	<ul><li>Reduced infection risk due to renal cysts</li><li>Eliminated risk of malignant transformation of renal cysts</li><li>Mechanical decompression</li><li>Free space for transplant kidney</li></ul>
Peri-Transplant	<ul><li>Longer surgical procedure</li><li>Increased blood loss</li><li>Prolonged anesthesia and related complications (DVT, atelectasis, etc.)</li><li>Increased risk of post-operative ileus</li><li>Possibility of intra-operative hypotension and hypo-perfusion of the graft kidney</li><li>Delay in kidney transplantation with prolonged CIT</li><li>Cancellation of kidney transplant due to patient instability during nephrectomy</li></ul>	<ul><li>Single surgical procedure</li><li>No requirement for dialysis</li></ul>
Post-Transplant	<ul><li>Increased risk of infections</li><li>Mechanical compression of native kidneys to allograft</li><li>Increased risk of Incisional hernia and wound dehiscence</li></ul>	<ul><li>Preservation of residual urine</li><li>No requirement for dialysis</li><li>Undergoing operation with stable transplant kidney function</li></ul>

Multiorgan Transplantation

The estimated prevalence of hepatic cysts in ADPKD patients is as high as 80% [24]. Liver involvement in ADPKD does not cause hepatic dysfunction. However, complications may develop due to increasing cyst sizes and infections. Complications of liver cysts continue even after patients develop ESRD and receive a kidney transplant. Hepatic lobe resection or liver transplantation may be considered in symptomatic patients who do not benefit from medical therapy. However, transplantation for polycystic liver disease is controversial, as liver function remains preserved until a late stage.

As with isolated liver transplantation, successful concurrent kidney-liver transplantations have been reported in a small number of patients. The choice of isolated liver transplantation or combined liver and kidney transplantation depends on pre-transplant kidney function. If liver transplantation is required in a dialysis-dependent ADPKD patient, a combined kidney and liver transplantation procedure has a distinct advantage [25].

Use of ADPBH Kidneys As Donor Kidney

Kidneys from donors affected by autosomal dominant polycystic kidney disease (ADPKD) are generally not suitable for transplantation. A limited number of transplants have been performed using cadaveric kidneys affected by ADPKD. Normally functioning cadaveric donor kidneys that show signs of early ADPKD, when implanted at an early stage of the disease, can function for years despite the progression of the cystic disease. In two separate studies with a 10-year and 15-year follow-up period, such an allograft had excellent function during follow-ups [26, 27].

REFERENCES

[1] Torres A. N. D. Harris P. C., Pirson Y.: Autosomal dominant polycystic kidney disease. *Lancet* 2007;369:1287-1301.
[2] Güler S., Çimen S., Hurton S., Molinari M.: Diagnosis and Treatment Modalities of Symptomatic Polycystic Kidney Disease. *Polycystic Kidney Disease* 2015; 978-0-9944381-0-2.
[3] Anafarta K., A. N., Bedük Y.: *Cystic Diseases of the Kidney in Basic Urology* 2011, Güneş Medical Bookstores: Ankara. p. 489-93.
[4] Fouad T. Chebib, MD and Vicente E. Torres, MD, PhD: Autosomal Dominant Polycystic Kidney Disease: *Core Curriculum* 2016.
[5] Hajj P.; Ferlicot S.; Massoud W.; Awad A.; Hammoudi Y.; Charpentier B.; Durrbach A.; Droupy S.; Benoit G. Prevalence of renal cell carcinoma in patients with autosomal dominant polycystic kidney disease and chronic renal failure. *Urology* 2009, 74, 631–634.
[6] Milutinovic J., Rust P. F., Fialkow P. J., et al.: Intrafamilial phenotypic expression of autosomal dominant polycystic kidney disease. *Am. J. Kidney Dis.* 1992; 19: pp. 465-472.
[7] Nicolau C., Torra R., Badenas C., Vilana R., Bianchi L., Gilabert R., Darnell A., Brú C.: Autosomal dominant polycystic kidney disease types 1 and 2: assessment of US sensitivity for diagnosis. *Radiology*. 1999 Oct; 213(1):273-6.
[8] Pirson Y., Chauveau D., Torres V.: Management of cerebral aneurysms in autosomal dominant polycystic kidney disease. *J. Am. Soc. Nephrol.* 2002;13:269-76.
[9] Ahsan Alam 1, Ronald D. Perroneİ: *Management of ESRD in patients with autosomal dominant polycystic kidney disease*, 2010 Mar; 17(2):164-72.
[10] Bretagnol Anne, Matthias Büchler, Jean-Michel Boutin, Hubert Nivet, Yvon Lebranchu, Dominique Chauveau : Renal transplantation in patients with autosomal dominant polycystic kidney disease: pre-transplantation evaluation and follow-up. *Nephrol. Ther.* 2007 Dec; 3(7):449-55. doi: 10.1016/j.nephro. 2007.07.002. Epub 2007 Sep 4.

[11] Mc Cune T. R., Nylander W. A., Van Buren D. H, Richie R. E., MacDonell R. C., Johnson H. K., et al.: Colonic screening prior to renal transplantation and its impact on posttransplant colonic complications. *Clin. Transplant.* 1992;6:91–6.

[12] Argyrou C., Moris D., Vernadakis S.: Tailoring the 'Perfect Fit' for Renal Transplant Recipients with End-stage Polycystic Kidney Disease: Indications and Timing of Native Nephrectomy. *In Vivo.* 2017 May-Jun; 31(3): 307–312.

[13] Bennett A. H., Stewart W., Lazarus J. M.: Bilateral nephrectomy in patients with polycystic renal disease. *Surg. Gynecol. Obstet.* 1973 Nov; 137(5):819-20.

[14] Wolfe, R. A.; Ashby, V. B.; Milford, E. L.; Ojo, A. O.; Ettenger, R. E.; Agodoa, L. Y.; Held, P. J.; Port, F. K. Comparison of mortality in all patients on dialysis, patients on dialysis awaiting transplantation, and recipients of a first cadaveric transplant. *N. Engl. J. Med.* 1999, 341, 1725–1730.

[15] Rayner B. L, Cassidy M. J. D., Jacobsen J. E.: Is preliminary binephrectomy necessary in patients with autosomal dominant polycystic kidney disease undergoing renal transplantation? *Clin. Nephrol.* 34:122, 1990.

[16] Meier-Kriesche H. U, Kaplan B.: Waiting time on dialysis as the strongest modifiable risk factor for renal transplant outcomes: A paired donor kidney. *Transplantation.* 2002;74(10):1377–1381.

[17] Abecassis M., Bartlett S. T., Collins A. J., Davis C. L., Delmonico F. L., Friedewald J. J., Hays R., Howard A., Jones E., Leichtman A. B, Merion R. M., Metzger R. A., Pradel F., Schweitzer E. J., Velez R. L., Gaston R. S.: Kidney transplantation as primary therapy for end-stage renal disease: A National Kidney Foundation/Kidney Disease Outcomes Quality Initiative (NKF/KDOQITM) conference. *Clin. J. Am. Soc. Nephrol.* 2008;3(2):471–480.

[18] Glassman D. T., Nipkow L., Bartlett S. T., Jacobs S. C.: Bilateral nephrectomy with concomitant renal graft transplantation for autosomal dominant polycystic kidney disease. *J. Urol.* 2000;164(3 Pt 1):661–664.

[19] Patel P., Horsfield C., Compton F., Taylor J., Koffman G., Olsburgh J.: Native nephrectomy in transplant patients with autosomal dominant polycystic kidney disease. *Ann. R. Coll. Surg. Engl.* 2011;93(5):391–395.

[20] Kirkman M. A., van Dellen D., Mehra S., Campbell B. A., Tavakoli A., Pararajasingam R., Parrott N. R., Riad H. N., McWilliam L., Augustine T.: Native nephrectomy for autosomal dominant polycystic kidney disease: Before or after kidney transplantation. *BJU Int.* 2011;108(4): 590–594.

[21] Lucas S. M., Mofunanya T. C., Goggins W. C., Sundaram C. P.: Staged nephrectomy versus bilateral laparoscopic nephrectomy in patients with autosomal dominant polycystic kidney disease. *J. Urol.* 2010 Nov; 184(5):2054-9.

[22] Ismail H. R., Flechner S. M., Kaouk J. H., Derweesh I. H., Gill I. S., Modlin C., Goldfarb D., Novick A. C.: Simultaneous vs. sequential laparoscopic bilateral native nephrectomy and renal transplantation. *Transplantation.* 2005 Oct 27; 80(8):1124-7.

[23] Gurung, P. M. S.; Frye, T. P.; Rashid, H. H.; Joseph, J. V.; Wu, G. Robot-assisted Synchronous Bilateral Nephrectomy for Autosomal Dominant Polycystic Kidney Disease: A Stepwise Description of Technique. *Urology* 2020.

[24] Bae K. T., Zhu F, Chapman A. B., vd.: Renal structure in early autosomal-dominant polycystic kidney disease (ADPKD): The Consortium for Radiologic Imaging Studies of Polycystic Kidney Disease (CRISP) cohort, *Clin. J. Am. Soc.. Nephrol.*, 2006, cilt. 1 (sf. 64-69).

[25] Ueno T., Barri Y. M., Netto G. J., et al.: Liver and kidney transplantation for polycysticliver and kidney-renal function and outcome. *Transplantation* 82:501-507, 2006.

[26] Eng M. K., Zorn K. C., Harland R. C., et al.: Fifteen-year follow-up of transplantation of a cadaveric polycystic kidney: A case report. *Transplant. Proc.* 2008; 40: pp. 1747-1750.
[27] Powell, C. R. 1, S. Tata, M. V. Govani, G. W. Chien, M. A. Orvieto, A. L. Shalhav: Transplantation of a cadaveric polycystic kidney in a patient with autosomal dominant polycystic kidney disease: long-term outcome. *Transplant. Proc.* 2004 Jun;36(5):1288-92.

INDEX

A

age, 6, 7, 12, 13, 14, 19, 36, 40, 48, 72, 80, 84, 86, 87, 88
anxiety, 39, 42, 43, 49, 50
arterial hypertension, 87
assessment, 35, 36, 37, 41, 45, 47, 50, 95
autosomal dominant, vii, 86, 94, 95, 96, 97, 98
awareness, 38, 46, 49

B

behavioral problems, viii, 33
beneficial effect, 10, 12, 17
bilateral, 80, 90, 91, 92, 97
biopsy, 6, 8, 15
bisphosphonate treatment, 17
bleeding, ix, 65, 67, 68, 84, 86, 88, 90, 91
blood, 3, 19, 64, 71, 72, 88, 91, 92, 93
blood flow, 3
blood pressure, 19, 73
blood supply, 71
blood transfusions, 88, 91

bone, vii, 1, 2, 3, 4, 5, 6, 7, 8, 9, 11, 13, 15, 16, 17, 18, 19, 20, 21
bone form, 6, 18
bone resorption, 2, 17
bone volume, 6, 7

C

calcification, 3, 9, 16, 19, 20
calcium, viii, 1, 2, 3, 4, 5, 6, 8, 9, 12, 16, 17, 18, 21
calcium-phosphorus metabolism, viii, 1, 2, 3, 10, 21
candidates, 34, 41, 50, 75, 88, 92
carbon dioxide, 67
cardiovascular risk, 73
cardiovascular system, 73
cholecalciferol, 9, 11, 16
chronic allograft rejection, viii, 34
chronic diseases, viii, 33, 34, 38
chronic illness, 38
chronic kidney disease, vii, viii, 1, 2, 3, 13, 21, 22, 24, 25, 27, 28, 30, 31, 33, 60
chronic renal failure, 39, 40, 87, 95
cognitive dysfunction, 49

cognitive function, 37
cognitive impairment, 40
compliance, vii, viii, 34, 35, 36, 37, 38, 39, 42, 48, 50
complications, vii, 6, 7, 18, 38, 40, 48, 49, 64, 65, 67, 69, 71, 73, 74, 77, 82, 87, 89, 90, 91, 92, 93, 94, 96
comprehension, 35, 44, 46
compression, ix, 84, 86, 88, 90, 93
computed tomography, 15, 87
controversial, 12, 15, 21, 92, 94
coronary heart disease, 20
cortical bone, 14, 16
cosmetic, 62, 64, 66, 76
cost, viii, ix, 18, 39, 61, 62, 70, 76

D

depression, 38, 39, 42, 43, 49
depressive symptoms, 39, 49
detection, 19, 35, 75
diabetes, viii, 1, 6, 7, 11, 14, 19, 34, 46, 72
diagnostic criteria, 88
dialysis, 5, 6, 7, 9, 10, 12, 13, 14, 19, 21, 36, 47, 48, 72, 90, 91, 93, 94, 96
diseases, viii, 33, 50, 73, 84, 88
disorder, ix, 4, 6, 7, 42, 83
donor nephrectomy, v, vii, ix, 51, 61, 62, 63, 64, 65, 66, 67, 68, 69, 70, 71, 72, 73, 74, 75, 76, 77, 78, 79, 80, 81, 82
donors, vii, viii, ix, 43, 44, 45, 46, 47, 49, 61, 62, 63, 67, 71, 72, 73, 74, 75, 76, 77, 80, 81, 82, 84, 88, 94
drug side effects, 48
drugs, 35, 49

E

economic well-being, 38
endocrine system, 73
endothelial cells, 20

end-stage renal disease, ix, 81, 83, 84, 96
evidence, 8, 10, 44, 79

F

family history, 14, 88, 89
family members, 44
family relationships, 44, 45
fascia, 63, 64, 65, 67, 70
feelings, 44, 46, 48, 49
financial, 43, 44, 45, 46
flank, ix, 61, 62, 63, 64, 78, 86
formation, 4, 6, 17, 68, 86, 89

G

guidelines, vii, viii, 2, 5, 6, 8, 10, 14, 15, 16, 19, 34, 41, 42, 81
guilt, 44, 46, 48, 49

H

health, vii, 1, 2, 4, 6, 11, 15, 19, 20, 37, 43, 45, 46, 50, 73
health effects, 45
health insurance, 46
history, ix, 4, 14, 37, 45, 62, 67, 89
hypercalcemia, 6, 8, 12, 16, 17, 18
hyperkalemia, 91, 93
hyperparathyroidism, 5, 6, 7, 8, 11, 12, 13, 14, 16, 17, 18
hyperphosphatemia, 4, 9, 16
hypertension, 34, 46, 72, 74, 81, 84, 86, 90
hypophosphatemia, 8, 12, 13, 16, 17

I

iliac crest, ix, 84, 89
immunomodulatory, 11
Immunosuppressants, 52

immunosuppressive agent, viii, 1, 11, 19
immunosuppressive drugs, 49
incidence, 8, 11, 14, 15, 16, 17, 18, 19, 20, 74
incisional hernia, 64, 68, 91
individuals, 38, 39, 42, 44, 50, 73, 75, 88
infection, 11, 35, 39, 48, 73, 86, 91, 93
injury, iv, 18, 65, 68, 81
intracranial aneurysm, 87, 89
ischemia, 64, 66, 68, 71, 80, 91
issues, vii, viii, 34, 37, 38, 88, 91

K

kidney, v, vii, viii, ix, 1, 2, 3, 5, 10, 12, 13, 15, 21, 22, 23, 24, 25, 26, 27, 28, 29, 30, 31, 33, 34, 35, 37, 39, 43, 44, 47, 48, 49, 50, 51, 52, 53, 54, 55, 56, 58, 59, 60, 62, 63, 64, 65, 67, 68, 69, 70, 71, 72, 74, 75, 76, 77, 78, 80, 81, 82, 83, 84, 86, 87, 88, 89, 90, 91, 92, 93, 94, 95, 96, 97, 98
kidney transplantation, v, vii, viii, ix, 1, 2, 4, 12, 15, 22, 24, 26, 27, 28, 29, 31, 33, 34, 35, 36, 39, 47, 51, 52, 54, 55, 58, 72, 80, 81, 84, 87, 89, 90, 92, 93, 94, 96, 97

L

liver, 11, 14, 47, 81, 84, 94
liver disease, 14, 94
liver donor, 47, 54
liver transplant, 81, 94
liver transplantation, 81, 94

M

malnutrition, 7, 14, 18
management, x, 41, 50, 84
medical, vii, 34, 35, 36, 37, 38, 39, 42, 44, 45, 46, 50, 94

mellitus, viii, 1, 13, 14
mental health, 43, 45
mental illness, 37, 39, 42, 50
meta-analysis, 68, 78, 81, 92
metabolism, viii, 1, 2, 3, 4, 10, 11, 13, 21
mineral bone disease, vii, 1, 2, 3, 4, 5, 8, 13, 21
minimally invasive surgical procedures, 62
morbidity, vii, 1, 2, 4, 73, 77, 82, 84
mortality, vii, 1, 2, 4, 6, 12, 13, 19, 39, 72, 74, 77, 81, 84, 89, 90, 96
mortality rate, 72, 89
mortality risk, 74

N

negative outcomes, 81
nephrectomy, v, vii, ix, 61, 62, 63, 64, 65, 66, 67, 68, 69, 70, 71, 73, 74, 75, 76, 77, 78, 79, 80, 81, 82, 83, 84, 86, 89, 90, 91, 92, 93, 96, 97

O

obesity, ix, 11, 62, 73, 81
obsessive-compulsive disorder, 42
organ, 34, 36, 39, 40, 44, 45, 47, 57, 59, 62, 70, 75, 76, 81, 82
osteodystrophy, 7, 93
osteoporosis, 7, 14, 18

P

pain, 8, 62, 64, 76, 77, 86, 90
pathology, vii, 1, 2, 4, 7, 9, 20
personality, 35, 36, 38, 39, 46, 48
personality disorder, 35, 39
personality traits, 38, 46, 48
phosphate, 3, 4, 5, 6, 8, 10, 12, 16, 17
phosphorus, viii, 1, 2, 13, 21

polycystic, v, vii, ix, 83, 84, 86, 87, 89, 91, 94, 95, 96, 97, 98
polycystic kidney disease, vii, ix, 83, 86, 89, 94, 95, 96, 97, 98
population, viii, ix, 2, 6, 11, 13, 14, 15, 16, 18, 19, 75, 83, 87, 88
post-transplant, viii, 1, 2, 6, 11, 12, 13, 14, 15, 16, 17, 18, 19, 20, 21, 34, 35, 37, 38, 39, 40, 47, 49, 50, 72, 89, 91
psychiatric disorder, 36, 37, 42
psychiatric illness, 42, 45, 49
psychiatrist, vii, viii, 34, 36, 37, 40, 43, 45, 48, 50
psychological evaluation, viii, 34, 36
psychological problems, 35
psychosocial factors, 35

Q

quality of life, viii, ix, 38, 39, 40, 47, 61, 62, 65, 70, 72, 75, 84, 90

R

renal cell carcinoma, 87, 95
renal failure, ix, 73, 74, 83, 84
renal osteodystrophy, 7, 9, 91
renal replacement therapy, 7
renal transplantation, viii, 17, 19, 21, 27, 41, 42, 55, 57, 61, 62, 72, 73, 75, 76, 78, 80, 89, 92, 95, 96, 97
risk, vii, ix, 6, 7, 9, 11, 12, 13, 14, 15, 16, 17, 18, 19, 34, 37, 38, 39, 40, 41, 42, 43, 44, 46, 48, 50, 62, 64, 68, 70, 73, 74, 81, 89, 91, 93, 96
risk factors, 12, 14, 19, 34, 37, 39, 41, 42, 44, 46, 48, 73

S

social change, 36
social relations, 38
social relationships, 38
social support, 36, 37, 38, 40, 41, 42, 43, 49
substance abuse, 35, 37, 41, 42, 43, 44, 45, 49
supplementation, 9, 11, 12, 13, 16, 18, 20
surgical technique, vii, ix, 45, 61, 62, 74, 75, 79, 92
survival, viii, ix, 2, 6, 10, 11, 12, 21, 35, 39, 48, 61, 62, 65, 66, 70, 72, 75, 76, 80, 84, 87, 91
symptoms, ix, 36, 38, 39, 42, 49, 83, 86, 89, 90

T

techniques, vii, ix, 61, 62, 63, 64, 65, 66, 67, 68, 69, 70, 72, 73, 75, 79, 92
therapy, 5, 6, 8, 14, 15, 87, 91, 94, 96
thoughts, 37, 39, 42, 50
transplant, vii, viii, ix, 1, 2, 9, 10, 11, 12, 13, 15, 16, 17, 18, 19, 21, 34, 35, 36, 37, 39, 40, 41, 42, 43, 44, 45, 48, 49, 50, 77, 80, 84, 88, 89, 90, 91, 92, 93, 94, 96, 97
transplant recipients, vii, viii, 1, 10, 49, 92
transplantation, vii, viii, ix, x, 17, 19, 21, 34, 35, 36, 37, 38, 39, 40, 41, 42, 43, 48, 49, 50, 59, 61, 62, 70, 72, 73, 75, 76, 78, 80, 81, 84, 89, 90, 91, 92, 94, 95, 96, 97, 98
transplantion, 84
treatment, vii, viii, ix, 2, 6, 7, 8, 9, 10, 12, 13, 14, 16, 17, 18, 19, 20, 21, 33, 35, 36, 37, 38, 39, 42, 43, 46, 48, 50, 83, 84, 87, 92
trial, 16, 20, 77, 78, 79, 80
turnover, 5, 6, 7, 8, 15, 16

U

ultrasonography, 88
ureter, 64, 65, 67, 71, 91
urinary tract, 18, 86, 88, 90
urinary tract infection, 18, 86, 88, 90

V

vein, 64, 65, 67, 70, 71, 74

vitamin D, 3, 6, 10, 19
vitamin D deficiency, 6

W

World Health Organization, 73
worldwide, viii, ix, 33, 41, 83, 84
wound dehiscence, 93
wound healing, 91
wound infection, 68